Grass Roots Injury Prevention

AF324922

Praise for this book

'This book is sorely needed. It conveys the importance of injury prevention in an engaging way, taking the theory and translating it into everyday practice. Health workers worldwide will be able to use this book to persuade their communities of the need for changed practices and of the possibility of lives saved.'
Professor Leif Svanström, Chair, WHO Collaborating Centre on Community Safety Promotion, Karolinska Institutet, Stockholm

'Successful injury prevention ultimately can only be achieved by programmes at the grass roots level. Simple guidelines, easily understood, without too much theory, easy to read by the people at that level – all these are extremely important, and these are what this book provides.'
Dr Witaya Chadbunchachai, Director, WHO Collaborating Centre for Injury Prevention and Safety Promotion, Khon Kaen Regional Hospital, Thailand

Grass Roots Injury Prevention

A guide for field workers

Diana Samarakkody, Elizabeth Davis
and Rod McClure

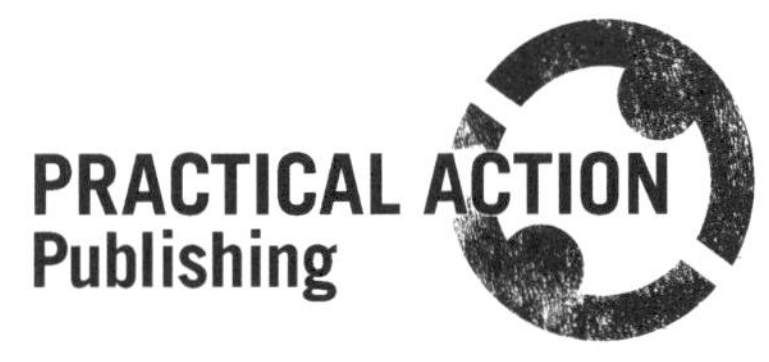

Practical Action Publishing Ltd
The Schumacher Centre
Bourton on Dunsmore, Rugby,
Warwickshire CV23 9QZ, UK
www.practicalactionpublishing.org

© Practical Action Publishing, 2013

ISBN 978-1-85339-802-5 Hardback
ISBN 978-1-85339-803-2 Paperback
ISBN 978-1-78044-802-2 Library Ebook
ISBN 978-1-78044-803-9 Ebook

Book DOI: http://dx.doi.org/10.3362/9781780448022

All rights reserved. No part of this publication may be reprinted or
reproduced or utilized in any form or by any electronic, mechanical, or
other means, now known or hereafter invented, including photocopying
and recording, or in any information storage or retrieval system, without
the written permission of the publishers.

A catalogue record for this book is available from the British Library.
The authors have asserted their rights under the Copyright Designs and
Patents Act 1988 to be identified as authors of this work.

Samarakkody, D., Davis, E., and McClure, R. (2013) *Grass Roots Injury
Prevention: A Guide for Field Workers*, Rugby, UK: Practical Action Publishing.

Since 1974, Practical Action Publishing has published and disseminated
books and information in support of international development work
throughout the world. Practical Action Publishing is a trading name of
Practical Action Publishing Ltd (Company Reg. No. 1159018), the wholly
owned publishing company of Practical Action. Practical Action Publishing
trades only in support of its parent charity objectives and any profits are
covenanted back to Practical Action
(Charity Reg. No. 247257, Group VAT Registration No. 880 9924 76).

Cover illustration by Susil Jayashantha Perera of Susil Sri Creations, Sri Lanka
Typeset by Bookcraft Limited, Stroud, Gloucestershire
Printed by Hobbs the Printers, United Kingdom

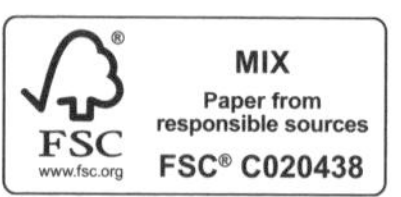

Contents

http://dx.doi.org/10.3362/9781780448022.000

Authors and contributors

About the authors

Dr Diana Samarakkody MBBS, MSc, MD is a Post-Doctoral Fellow, Monash University Accident Research Centre, Australia. She is a public health physician and injury epidemiologist. Diana is currently National Program Manager for Injury Prevention and Control in the Injury Prevention Division of the Ministry of Health, Sri Lanka. She is an adviser for the establishment of the first Safe Community in Sri Lanka, in the city of Horana. Diana is involved in multi-disciplinary research projects looking for solutions to the problem of injury and teaches injury prevention and management to undergraduate and postgraduate medical students. She is an accredited PhD supervisor at the Monash Injury Research Institute (MIRI), Monash University, Australia.

Elizabeth Davis GCert Mngt, is a Research Officer with Injury Prevention and Control (Australia) Ltd. She has a Graduate Certificate in Management and more than 20 years' experience in health promotion, health policy, and programme evaluation. Elizabeth's specific expertise lies in the social determinants of health and applying this expertise to project planning, implementation and evaluation at all levels. In 2000, she received the Queensland Director-General's Excellence in Health Services Delivery Award for a project she devised and implemented called 'Safety in Residential Dwellings: increasing safety devices and features in the home'.

Professor Rod McClure MBBS, BA, PhD, FAFPHM, FAICD is Director, Monash Injury Research Institute (MIRI) and Professor, Faculty of Medicine, Nursing and Health Sciences, Monash University, Australia; Adjunct Professor, Institute for Social and Health Studies, University of South Africa, Johannesburg, South Africa. He has medical qualifications, extensive clinical experience in emergency medicine, a PhD in injury epidemiology, and specialist training in public health medicine. Rod received the Australian 2009 Special Award for Excellence in Injury Prevention/Safety Promotion Research and the 2011 Research Award from the Australian Injury Prevention Network. He is on the editorial board of the *Journal of Injury Prevention* and the *Journal of Health and Safety Research & Practice*, and is editor of two books and author of more than 120 peer-reviewed journal articles on injury prevention. Rod has been a member of the International Organizing Committee for the World Conferences on Injury Prevention and Safety Promotion since 2010.

About the contributors

Professor Samath Dharmaratne MBBS, MSc, MD is Head of the Department of Community Medicine, Faculty of Medicine, University of Peradeniya, Sri Lanka; an Associate Professor in Community Medicine; and a Consultant Community Physician. He is a Senior Fellow of the Postgraduate Institute of Medicine, University of Colombo, Sri Lanka, and an Affiliate Assistant Professor at the Institute for Health Metrics and Evaluation, University of Washington, United States. Samath has been involved in injury prevention, especially road injury prevention, for the past 15 years in Sri Lanka and the region.

Professor Mohamed Seedat DPhil is Head of the Institute for Social and Health Sciences at the University of South Africa and Director of the Safety and Peace Promotion Research Unit, a partnership between the South African Medical Research Council and the University of South Africa. Mohamed's research interests include violence and injury prevention, safety and peace promotion, the politics of knowledge production, as well as the role of spirituality and religion in human development.

Sherianne Kramer MA (Hons), BADA is a registered South African research psychologist at the University of South Africa Institute for Social and Health Sciences. Her responsibilities include coordination of community-level data collection, and the analysis, interpretation and reporting of results. Sherianne's research interests include crime, violence and injury prevention, female sex crimes, gender performativity and knowledge production. Her PhD research explores the issue of sexual assault by women.

Preface

Everyone in a community is affected when someone dies or is disabled by an injury. Children lose a parent; families have to care for an injured loved one, sometimes for many years; the community loses people who could have contributed to its prosperity and wellbeing.

Injury accounts for 9 per cent of global mortality and 90 per cent of these deaths occur in lower- and middle-income countries. As countries become more industrialized and motorized, the burden of injury is expected to grow.

It is possible to prevent injuries that kill and disable. The cost of *not* preventing these injuries is high.

Grass Roots Injury Prevention: A Guide for Field Workers (henceforth called *The GRIP Guide*) will help field workers who want to help make their communities safer.

Books on injury prevention are often written by authors who come from academia and seldom consider the challenges and everyday realities faced by the field worker. The books tend to explain the principles and leave it to the practitioner to work out how to apply them. *The GRIP Guide* aims to bridge the gap between 'what works in principle' and 'what works in practice'. It is designed to be used in everyday situations, not left on a shelf as a reference.

The authors have assumed that readers have a sound education and a basic understanding of many of the terms commonly used in injury prevention. Those who want more detailed information about the theory and models underpinning injury prevention and safety promotion are encouraged to read the companion book, *The Scientific Basis of Injury Prevention and Control* (McClure et al., 2004).

Acknowledgements

We thank Jill Henry for suggesting we write this book and encouraging us to persevere until it was done. Inspiration for the approach we have taken in this book was drawn from two publications, *Training for Transformation* by Anne Hope and Sally Timmel and *Where There Is No Doctor* by David Werner. We thank these authors for their insights. For the wonderful illustrations, we thank Susil Jayashantha Perera, of Susil Sri Creations, Sri Lanka. We especially thank Anne Burgi, of SUBStitution Pty Ltd, for helping us edit the text to fit its intended function.

Part I

CHAPTER 1
Introduction to *The GRIP Guide*

Injuries are a leading cause of death and disability for all age groups, among all people, in all parts of the world. Yet injuries are one of the most preventable health conditions we face. Grass Roots Injury Prevention: A Guide for Field Workers *has been written for field workers who want to help make their communities safer.* The GRIP Guide *translates the principles of injury prevention into everyday practice. It helps you understand what causes injuries and what can be done to prevent them.*

Keywords: injury prevention, guide, manual, field workers

Who it will help

If you are working to prevent injuries and promote safety at individual, family, and village levels in lower- and middle-income countries, *The GRIP Guide* is for you!

Community health workers are looking for simple, effective ways to prevent injuries and promote safety. This is a practical manual to help you make a difference, without the need to wade through the theory of individual, social, and environmental change that underpins injury prevention and safety promotion.

How to use it

The GRIP Guide is designed to help translate the principles of injury prevention into everyday practice. It will help readers understand what causes injuries and what can be done to prevent them. It takes into account the human, social, environmental, and financial challenges in many communities. The book focuses on preventing the causes of injury (primary prevention).

The GRIP Guide provides a series of approaches community health workers can use to help ordinary people create safer homes, villages and communities. The explanation of these approaches is based on the experiences of a fictional field worker named Dula and a

http://dx.doi.org/10.3362/9781780448022.001

group of community members in the fictional village of Dingly. The exercises provide community health workers with tools they can use to bring community leaders and members together to identify the main causes of injury and propose lasting solutions that will work in their community.

Readers can select the modules (sections) that reflect the types of injuries in their communities. Each module provides the information that community members and leaders need to help them take action.

The GRIP Guide does not provide a blueprint for you to simply copy. Instead, it provides a process to help you guide the community in developing the answers for themselves. *The GRIP Guide* helps you 'learn by doing', not 'do by copying'.

We recommend you read the whole manual carefully to enable you to understand the purpose, content, and approach taken. To help others to learn and to act in their own communities, you must be familiar with the key information provided in each exercise.

The guide will help you help others – such as community members and leaders or key decision-makers in schools, workplaces, and government departments – to understand the major causes of injuries, and what they can do to build and maintain safe places for people to live, work, and play.

At the end of each exercise, the guide encourages you to think of other possibilities and alternative ways to address the problem under discussion.

How it is structured

The GRIP Guide contains seven modules following the introductory chapters.

Chapter 2 gives an overview of the principles of injury prevention and safety promotion. Modules 1 to 5 describe how to address the five main types of unintentional injuries (burns, falls, drowning, transport injuries, poisoning). Module 6 describes an approach to preventing intentional injuries (violence). Module 7 provides a generic approach to reducing the risk of other unintentional injuries.

These modules can be used flexibly; you do not need to follow the sequence from 1 through to 7. The authors encourage you to read all modules as each provides information of value to you in working toward lasting change. However, you can choose to focus on the module about the injury of most concern to your community. *The GRIP Guide* is there to support you and your community to learn through doing.

Each module is designed to help build confidence and skills in:

- Grasping the problem;
- Risk factor identification;
- Intervention development and implementation;
- Progress monitoring.

INTERVENTION

An intervention is a planned activity that is designed to prevent injury. For example, building a childproof fence around a well is an intervention to prevent children drowning. An effective intervention is purposeful and combines a number of ways (strategies) to remove the things (risk factors) known to cause injury. You will learn more about how to develop interventions and put them into practice as you go through *The GRIP Guide*.

Making *The GRIP Guide* work for you

To improve the local relevance of the exercises provided, you may wish to use local names and local stories. Carefully consider any cultural and religious issues that are important to your community when adapting the exercises. You also need to think about the financial, physical, or geographic restrictions that may make an exercise difficult in your community.

One person cannot have all the knowledge, skills and authority to change many of the factors that cause injury. We recommend you seek the assistance and support of local officials and community members each step of the way, from gathering information about the problem through to putting lasting solutions in place.

How to form a group

To get the most out of *The GRIP Guide*, you will need to work with a wide range of people. Bringing them together in a group will enable you to build on their experience and skills. Forming a group involves getting together people who share an interest in an area (such as injury prevention) or who have responsibility for the things found to be causing injuries, and who are prepared to work with others to achieve the community's goals.

Begin by identifying the most senior members of the community, such as elders, the chief priest, political leaders, business owners, aid organization representatives, police, and medical and nursing professions in the village. Arrange to visit each of these people to talk about the problem of injury in your community. Ask them to support your plan to establish a group to work on ways to reduce injuries in the community. Present them with a summary of the problem of injury in your community and some of the ways the community could be made safer. Explain how improved safety would be good for the community, the government, and businesses.

When arranging meetings find a time when most people will be available, considering work, family and community commitments, and then provide everyone with details of where and when the first meeting will be held. At that first meeting, you can help those present discuss how the group will function in the future.

Learning exercises

Group exercises and various activities are used to encourage community members and leaders to take part. The following pages describe these activities.

Brainstorming

Brainstorming helps people work together to build a solution to a problem. The group members' experiences, skills, and knowledge of their own community can lead to new approaches to removing a problem.

Steps

- Write the problem on a flipchart or blackboard. For example: what can we do to prevent burn injuries in the village?
- Ask group members to think about the problem for a few minutes.

- Encourage them to put forward their ideas.
- Write all the ideas on the board as they are mentioned. Do not interrupt or argue; let the ideas flow freely. It is important to record all the ideas – no matter how unusual or unlikely to work they may seem to you. If there appear to be any areas of confusion, encourage everyone to explain their ideas a bit more.
- Work with the group members to allocate the ideas to themes such as 'in the home'; 'in the workplace'; 'in the village'.
- With the group members, consider how often the injury happens and its severity. Prioritize the ideas within each group according to the urgency for action. Ask the questions: What must we do now? What can we do over the next three months? What do we need to do in the future?

Case study

A case study is a detailed story – real or made up – about an event that led to one or more injuries. It enables group members to realize that their families and community members may be at risk of similar injuries. Encourage the group members to think about what was happening when the injury took place, what caused the injury, and what action could have prevented the injury from happening.

If you use a real story, change the names of people and the community described in the story to protect their privacy. It is important to make sure that no hurt can be done through the telling of a story in which a loved one might be easily identified.

Steps

- Divide your group into smaller teams of three or four members. Bigger teams can make it difficult for everyone to be heard.
- Give each team a copy of the case study (e.g. a detailed story about an event resulting in burns to a three-year-old child).
- Ask team members to read and discuss the case study. You may need to prompt the discussion with some questions, such as: What are the main things you think contributed to the injury? What could have been done differently? What must happen to prevent a similar injury in our village?

- Bring the small teams back together to discuss all the ideas put forward.
- Write down the ideas on the board as they are mentioned.
- Work with the members to put the ideas into logical themes around the type of injury described in the case study, such as 'in the home'; 'in the workplace'; 'in the village'.
- Work with the group members to prioritize each idea under headings, such as 'What must we do now?'; 'What can we do over the next three months?'; 'What do we need to do in the future?'

Community mapping

Community mapping can be used to assess the potential risks to safety in places where the community members live, work, and play. Features mapped might include:

- natural landmarks, such as rivers, channels, wells, jungle, wild animal crossings;
- human-built structures, such as cooking areas, roads, livestock pens, and playing areas;
- common activities, such as farming, washing, and building.

Steps

- Have group members draw a map of their area on a large sheet of paper.
- Ask them to mark features that are important in relation to the problem being discussed. For example, if you are discussing drowning, mark all the wells and bodies of water.
- Ask them to describe any injuries that are related to these features.
- Discuss the relationships between the features on the map and the injuries that have occurred.
- Encourage group members to share their ideas about what could be done to reduce the risk of injuries in these areas in the future.

Daily activity schedule

Ask the group members to record their daily activities to help them identify behaviour that could place them or their loved ones at risk of an injury. Use this exercise when helping people understand that individual behaviour is an important factor in preventing injury.

Demonstrations

Demonstrations are a good way to give people a strong message. For example, setting alight a flammable item of children's clothing or seeing the damage done by falling building material will be more effective and leave a longer-lasting message than just describing it.

Steps

- Explain the purpose of the demonstration.
- Encourage group members to ask questions.
- Demonstrate the behaviour or other factors that could cause an injury.
- Ask group members to role-play (see below) the event.
- Discuss the feasibility, advantages, and disadvantages of reducing exposure to the things shown to be the causes of an injury.
- With the group members, explore how they could overcome any potential barriers to reducing these causes in their community.
- Encourage group members to make a list of actions under each of the headings: 'What must we do now?'; 'What can we do over the next three months?'; 'What do we need to do in the future?'

Event calendars and charts

Keeping event calendars and charts can provide information about the size of the injury problem in a community. They also help monitor the success of activities designed to reduce the risk or severity of injuries. Group members can be encouraged to record the details of injuries that occur in their village over several months or seasons. This will provide valuable information about the frequency, severity, and seasonal variation of injuries.

Group discussions

Group discussions encourage members to share their ideas and experiences. Open discussions help group members realize that they are better able to find ways to reduce the risk of injury in their village if they work together.

Steps

- Group discussions can be in small teams of three or four people or as a large group.
- Start by agreeing on the rules of the group discussion. Group rules might include:
    - listen to each other without interrupting;
    - respect each other's ideas, values, and beliefs;
    - do not insult or cause intentional hurt through negative comments, looks or gestures;
    - give views briefly, clearly, and keep discussions on the topic.
- To help give everyone an opportunity to join the discussion, you might use a 'talking stick' to identify the person who is speaking. This is a stick or similar object that is passed to each group member in turn to encourage them to share their ideas while everyone else listens.
- Select one person in the group to lead the discussion and, if necessary, to remind group members of the agreed rules.
- If the discussion is in smaller teams, ask each team to choose a member to present the summary of their discussion to the whole group. Encourage all group members to be involved in discussing each summary.

Field visits

Field visits provide group members with first-hand experience of where injuries happen.

Steps

- Decide on a place to visit that is relevant to the injury the group is focused on.

- If needed, plan safe transport and access to clean water, and organize meals for the day of the field visit.
- Think about the observations and activities that will increase the group's knowledge.
- Prepare a checklist for each group member, drawing attention to injury risk factors. The checklist should encourage them to look at the physical features, such as the layout of the site; the natural landmarks; the activities taking place; and who is involved in them.
- After the field visit, bring the group together to discuss their observations and experiences. Use the checklist to guide discussions about the site's features and people's behaviour that increased or decreased the risk of injury.

Folk media

Folk media (lullabies, nursery rhymes, folk songs, and puppets) can be used to convey important information about ways to stay safe and to prevent injuries among people of all ages and backgrounds.

Games

Games specific to a group's culture and community can support learning and help people to work together.

If the group members are not well known to each other, you might need to think of ways to 'break the ice' before people will join in or share their ideas. Group games specific to their culture may help everyone relax and be a more confident member of the group.

Presentations

Presentations by experts in a subject area can raise awareness within a community and increase knowledge about preventive actions.

Experts can come from many different places and backgrounds. They might include the local baby health nurse presenting practical ways to keep a baby safe; an officer from the Department of Agriculture demonstrating how to use farm chemicals safely; or the local doctor talking about what to do to reduce the skin damage if someone is scalded by hot water.

Presenters need to select information that will be meaningful to the group members, taking into account their level of education and any cultural issues that may influence their reactions.

Role play

Role play is an unrehearsed, unscripted drama in which group members act out an event. Role plays of injuries can motivate group members to change their behaviour to avoid injuries.

Steps

Choose a situation: for example, a fire caused by an overloaded power board breaks out in a home while the family is gathered to watch TV or an elderly grandmother is severely burnt while preparing the evening meal.

- Ask group members to select their roles and give them some time together to prepare (no script is needed; the 'actors' should make up their own words and actions).
- Ask them to act out what was happening before, during, and after the injury happened.
- Encourage the whole group to discuss the behaviour and features that could have contributed to causing, or increasing the severity of, the injury.

The learning environment

Having a good place to meet plays an important role in supporting people to learn about injury prevention and safety promotion. Consider the following:

- *The venue or location.* Choose a place where everyone feels emotionally and physically safe. This might be an auditorium, a community hall, a room in a group member's home, the lunch room at a factory, or in a shaded area outside. Most importantly, the venue must be free from noise and distractions such as children, traffic, or machinery. Where mobile phone use is common, remember to ask group members to switch them off before you start the meeting.

- *The facilities available in the venue.* Make sure you know what is and is not available, such as lighting, drinking water, sanitary facilities, ventilation, and access to electricity if using electronic resources.
- *Seating.* Interactive learning is best when all the group members are able to easily see and hear each other and the facilitator. Sitting in a circle, semicircle or horseshoe will allow all group members to be actively involved in discussions.
- *Notes.* People may want to take notes to help them remember all the information, so encourage one person to write the group's responses somewhere everyone can see. Invite the whole group to talk about the responses; talking about an idea can help people remember the information later.

Learning materials

Few resources are needed when using *The GRIP Guide,* but some suggestions are listed below.

- *Something to write the main information and messages on.* This can be as simple as a blank wall, floor or sand tray, or as formal as a blackboard, flipchart paper, large sheets of paper, whiteboards, or magnet boards. Things to remember:
    - allow time during or at the end of each session for group members to copy down the information;
    - where possible, let group members do the writing, as this encourages participation and ownership of the information;
    - encourage the use of large, clear, simple letters that allow all group members to read what has been suggested;
    - make sure that all the group members can see the writing;
    - if appropriate, give all group members a fact sheet clearly and simply describing and illustrating key information (using fact sheets can enable group members to join the discussions rather than being distracted by trying to take notes).
- *Something to write with, such as chalk, pens, markers, crayons, and sticks.* Avoid colours that cannot be read easily, such as yellow, pink, and orange. Red and green are also best avoided as some people are colour blind and cannot see these two colours clearly.

- *Materials for group members to take notes on, such as school exercise books or notebooks.* Writing down information can help reinforce learning. It also provides group members with a lasting resource that they can use themselves or to accurately share information with others.
- *Locally available publications.* Posters, leaflets, flash cards, and booklets published by health, education, and road departments, and police, can help start discussions about common injuries. Providing information in different formats can encourage people to think about the causes of injuries and ways to reduce the risk of them happening.
- *'People' resources.* Listening to the experiences of an injured person and their loved ones or those of members of local healthcare teams and the local fire brigade can motivate people to take action to prevent the risk of injuries.
- *Electronic resources,* such as videos and films, can help focus a group on an injury problem. These resources may be available in the local or mobile library or from local government departments.

Ethical issues

The GRIP Guide emphasizes the need to combine the best available evidence with local information to ensure that any interventions have the best chance to work. In many cases, local information is available in publicly available books and documents. However, if your group collects any data, it is vital that they consider the potential ethical issues arising from the collection of the data or its use. Remember the community owns any data you gather and must consent to how and where it is to be used.

It is assumed throughout this book that, where needed, ethics approval has been given by the relevant authorities. When you are following the examples provided in the book, check your local ethics approval and monitoring procedures before you begin.

It is essential the privacy of all those described in any data or case studies is protected at all times. No information can be provided that might make it possible for an individual, family or community to be identified unless they have given their full approval for its use.

Our success story

I created a number of 'hands-on' learning opportunities, including small group discussions, field visits, brainstorming sessions, case studies, demonstrations, and games. I designed learning activities with lots of drawings and minimal written materials. For most activities, I used locally available resources.

To increase awareness of the damage that injuries were doing to the lives and futures of people living in Dingly, the Injury Prevention Committee of Dingly organized workshops, festivals, competitions, street plays, and processions. We invited council members, religious leaders, government officers, business owners, representatives from non-government organizations (NGOs) to these activities.

This work strengthened the networks and relationships to unite people around a common issue. This led to more people across the community calling for action. Politicians advocated on our behalf to convince the national and regional governments to act to prevent injuries in Dingly.

As a result of our efforts, over time we dramatically reduced the number and severity of injuries in our community. We have learnt a lot and we will continue to learn as we evaluate how effective our activities have been.

I hope our experiences and the improvements we have achieved will stimulate your thoughts about establishing an injury prevention network to help make your community safe.

Yours sincerely,

Dula

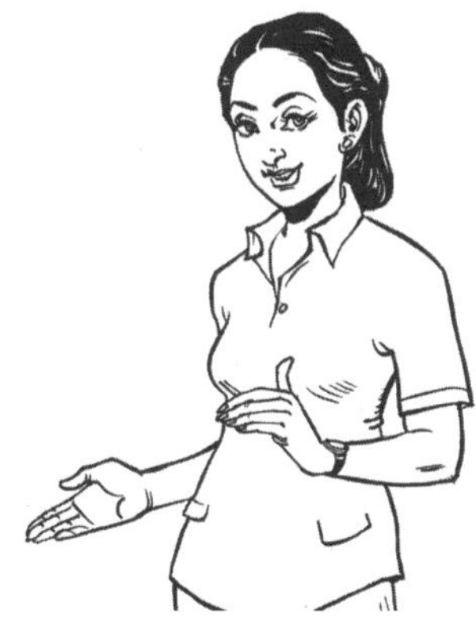

CHAPTER 2

Injury prevention and safety promotion

The process of injury control begins with describing the nature and extent of the problem of injury in your community. The next task for you as prevention practitioners is to identify the risk factors for injuries that are a problem in your community. Once you have done this you will be able to develop interventions to address the risk factors. These interventions are activities that can be undertaken throughout the whole of your community. Active monitoring of the success of your interventions completes the prevention cycle. Monitoring provides the information required to redefine the problem of injury in your community and lays the groundwork for further preventive efforts.

Keywords: surveillance, risk factors, interventions, action plans

Grasping the problem

What is injury?

During Dula's first weeks as a health worker in Dingly, she saw a lot of people hurt. It seemed that almost every day there was an injury that affected the lives of people in the village.

On the very first week, she went to the hospital to see Nagayya, who had been seriously injured by a wild elephant. Dula was also called to resuscitate a local fisherman named Abdul, who had been found floating in the river. Karishma's seven-year-old son, Ajey, had broken his forearm falling from a tree. Kumari, an epileptic mother of three children, had severe burns over her face and chest after falling onto an open fire while she was cooking.

Dula realized action must be taken. Her first step was to bring together a group of villagers and community leaders to talk about the problem. She asked them to describe the events they knew where someone was hurt and what these events had in common. She also asked them to think about what the word 'injury' meant to them.

http://dx.doi.org/10.3362/9781780448022.002

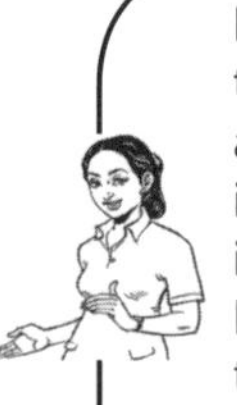

Bring together the people you think are best placed to help you tackle the problem of injury in your community. Once you have agreed on the group rules ask everyone to think about a recent injury in their community. Call on one or two to describe where the injury happened and what those involved were doing at the time. Let the discussion flow for 5–10 minutes and then bring the group together to summarize what they see as the main things common to all the stories. Then, ask a simple question: 'What is an injury?' Write down an answer that everyone agrees on.

Energy and injury

Dula explained to her group that things that move have energy. When moving things hit you, they pass that energy on to you. Hot water has energy: when it touches you, it passes the energy on to you. When there is not enough heat energy we get frostbite, or die of exposure. When we do not get enough oxygen we suffocate. When there is too much, or not enough energy, it damages us. We call that damage 'injury'. Dula demonstrated by striking a metal bar with a hammer. She asked them to feel the heat and the dent in the bar caused when the energy was transferred from her arm through the hammer to the bar.

It is important the group understands that the transfer of energy is the main factor leading to the damage that we call injury. This understanding will enable agreement on what action should be taken to prevent the injury.

INJURY

Injury is harm to the body caused by the sudden transfer of too much or too little energy.

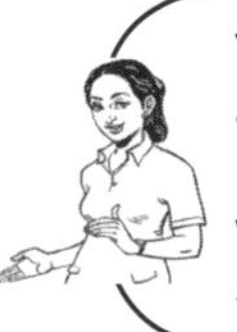

Your group will probably not use the word 'energy' when they talk about injury, but they may understand what Dula meant when she used the word. In the next exercise, your group will talk more about why 'energy' is such an important concept in injury prevention and safety promotion.

Dula asked the group to think of sources of energy that can cause an injury. Then she passed the 'talking stick' around the group so that all members could get a chance to tell about the energy sources they thought caused unintentional injuries.

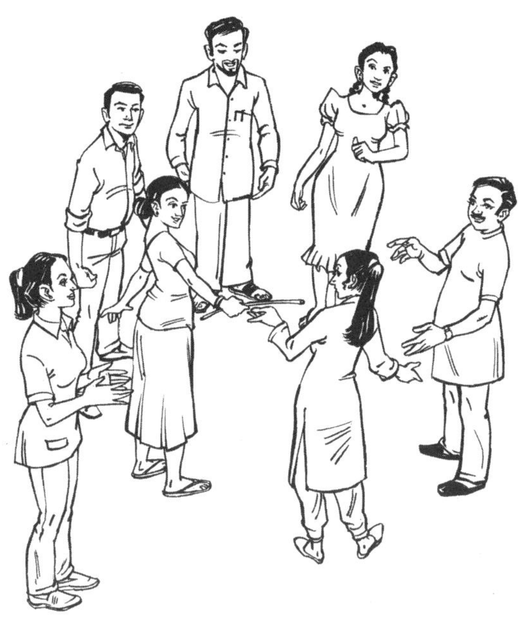

Dula's group identified the following energy sources that can harm the body:

- moving objects, such as a speeding motor vehicle or stampeding animals;
- blunt surfaces, such as low-hanging branches;
- cutting or piercing tools, such as harvesting knives, axes;
- explosive devices, such as landmines, bombs;
- poisons and other chemicals, such as battery acid, cleaning products;
- electrical equipment, such as household appliances, tools;
- fires;
- hot water;
- extreme cold;
- bodies of water;
- chemical fumes.

Types of energy

The above energy sources can be thought of in terms of:

- kinetic energy – energy transferred from:
  - moving objects;
  - sudden contact with a blunt surface;
  - sudden contact with a sharp surface;
  - explosive devices;
- chemical energy – transferred during contact with chemical substances;
- electrical energy – transferred during contact with electric current;
- heat – energy transferred during heating or cooling;
- oxygen – energy restricted by lack of access to oxygen such as when underwater.

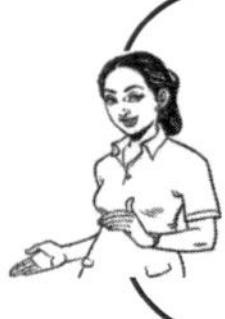

Ask your group to think of the types of energy that can harm the body. Write the group's ideas on a board or flipchart. How do the answers your group gave compare to the list that Dula's group wrote? Dula's list might give you some ideas you can discuss with your own group.

Types of injury

Dula's group brainstormed the types of injury that can occur when a person is suddenly exposed to too much or too little energy. Their responses were written on flipchart paper where all could read them. The list included:

- bruising;
- bleeding;
- cuts/lacerations;
- broken bones;
- crushing;
- puncture wounds;
- dislocation of joints;
- strains and sprains;
- scalds/burns.

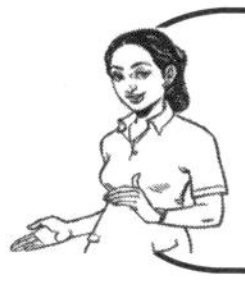

What body parts are damaged?

With the help of her group, Dula prepared a body-sized sheet of paper by pasting together smaller papers. She asked one of the group to lie on the paper while the others traced his outline.

The group members sat around the drawing and identified the parts of the body that can be damaged when a person is exposed to a transfer of too little or too much energy.

It became clear to Dula's group that all parts of the body can be injured.

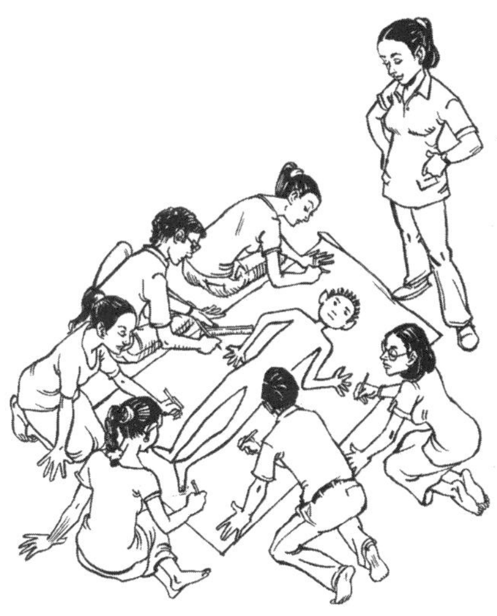

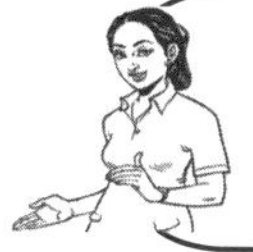

What is an injury event?

In most examples, Dula's group had described not only the injury itself but also where the injury happened and what people were doing at the time. Dula explained that it was useful to separate the idea of an 'injury' from the 'injury event' that leads to the injury.

The difference is that an 'injury' is the damage to the body caused by a sudden energy transfer. 'Injury events' are all the things that come together resulting in too much or too little energy being transferred. An 'injury event' will be explored later in the book.

What locations and activities are involved?

Dula divided her group into two teams and asked one team to call out the name of a place where an injury can happen, for example, 'Home'. The members of the other team described common activities at that location; for example, cooking, playing, washing, and gardening. Both teams then described injuries that are known to have happened while doing each activity.

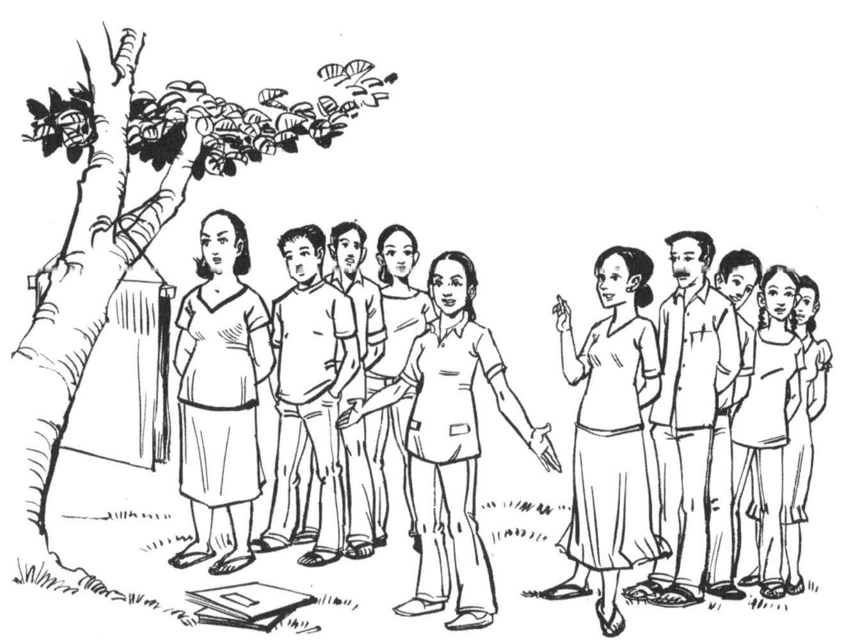

One group member wrote their responses on flipchart paper as shown in Table 2.1.

Table 2.1 Locations and activities in which injury can occur

Where?	What activity?
Home	Cooking, playing, repairing, washing, eating, cleaning
Garden	Mowing, trimming, digging
Workplace	Welding, cleaning, walking, climbing stairs, chopping, lifting
Farm	Puddling, harvesting, milling, packing
Playground	Running, jumping, swinging, sliding, climbing
Street	Walking, riding, driving
River	Swimming, bathing, fishing, boating, washing

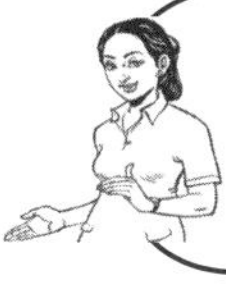

Follow Dula's example with your group to help them understand that an injury can occur anywhere and while doing almost all everyday activities.

What are injury outcomes?

After getting the permission of those involved, Dula wrote four short stories, each describing an injury event in Dingly over the past month. Dula divided her group into teams of three or four people and nominated a storyteller for each team. She gave each storyteller one of the stories to read to their group and asked them to discuss the story.

Dula put up some questions on the flipchart to encourage people to think about the full impact of the injury. Dula's questions were:

- What is the severity of the injury?
- What are the outcomes of the injury for:
    - the person?
    - the family members and loved ones?
    - the community?

Here are the stories Dula gave to her group to discuss.

Story 1

Seven-year-old Mohan was playing with his sister in the garden outside their house. He was climbing up onto a pile of old boxes when the boxes collapsed and he fell, breaking his arm as he landed on the hard ground.

Story 2

Kumari, an epileptic mother of three children, had run out of medicines several months earlier and had not taken any since. She had a seizure while cooking, causing the open stove to overturn when she fell. She suffered severe burns over her face and chest, and spent three weeks recovering in hospital.

Story 3

Nagayya was a 39-year-old farmer, with three preschool-aged children, who was crushed against a hut by a wild elephant storming through his farm. Nagayya suffered severe damage to both legs and has since been unable to stand for long periods. He is unlikely to walk properly again.

Story 4

Abdul, who could not swim, was going to the markets across the river in his boat heavily laden with coconut. The river current was strong and a strong wind was creating waves that overturned the boat. Michel, who was fishing nearby, jumped in and pulled Abdul out, but he died before Michel could carry him to the hospital.

Following the smaller team discussions, a member from each small team presented the summary of their discussion about the outcome of injuries. Dula's whole group then shared their views on the severity of injuries, and the impacts on the lives and future outcomes for both the injured person and their family members in each case study.

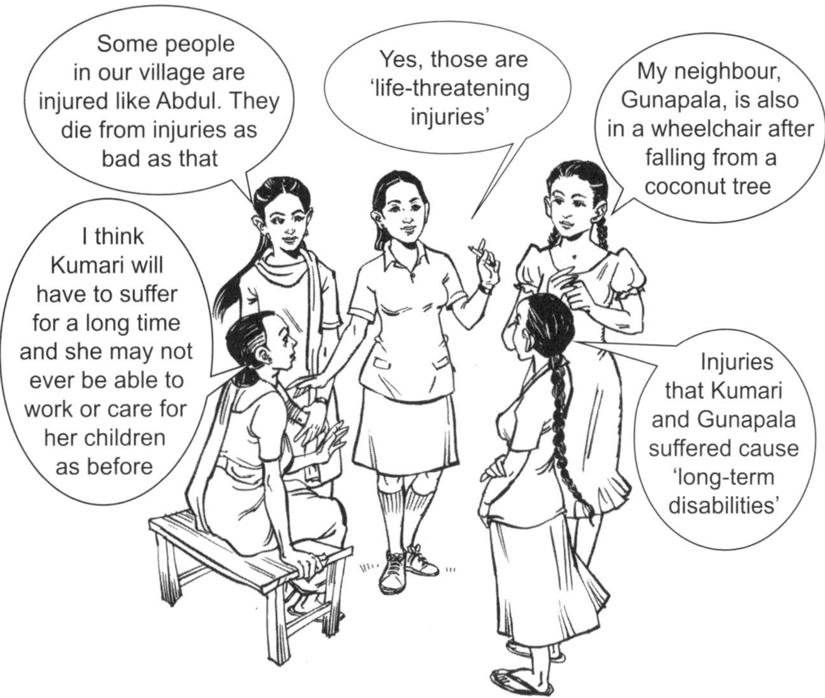

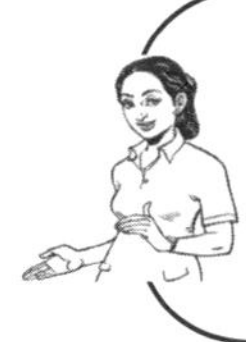

Dula's teams wrote the following possible outcomes on the flipchart.

Injured person

- pain;
- swelling;
- bleeding;
- not being able to move at all or moving less freely than before;
- scarring and disfigurement;
- loss of dreams and expectations of marriage and children;
- depression, anger or feelings of hopelessness;
- loss of school or working days;
- unemployment;

- inability to carry out duties in the family and the community;
- death.

Family members

- the cost to the family of paying for treatment;
- physical problems faced by the family trying to care for a severely injured person;
- loss of the family income;
- family members having to do the work in the home, farm or business usually done by the injured person.

Community

- the cost of providing trauma and hospital care;
- the cost of providing rehabilitation and support services;
- loss of income to business owners due to the loss or reduced output of a skilled worker;
- loss of income to the shopkeepers and tradespeople because the injured person and their family have less to spend;
- the injured person and their family members not making their usual contribution to the social and cultural life of the community.

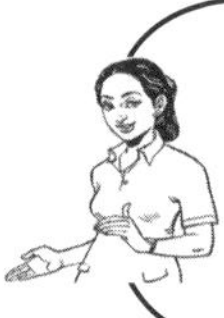

Ask your teams to make a similar list. At the end of the discussions bring the group together to summarize what they found to be the main outcomes for the injured person, their family, and their community. They should think about not only the physical and emotional outcomes soon after the injury, but also the outcomes into the future.

How arc injuries caused?

Dula used a set of questions on the blackboard to help her group find out more about the injuries in Dingly:

1. What was the type of energy involved?
2. When was the energy released/transferred?
3. What happened during the event to make this energy transfer occur?
4. What things shaped the way the injury occurred?
5. What could have been done to prevent the injury from happening?

These concepts were not easy to explain, but Dula knew that if the group did not understand what things contribute to an injury, they would not be able to work out what actions were needed to reduce the causes of injury in Dingly.

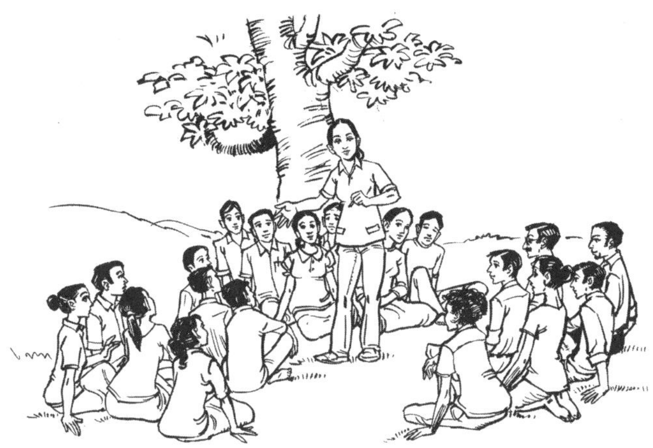

Dula talked about factors that could be identified as causes at the individual and family levels. She showed how they were different from the causes of injury at the community/neighbourhood and population levels.

Through field visits and group discussions, her group saw that the things they had identified as causes of injuries were common in areas used every day by the people of Dingly. The group came to understand these as risk factors. They recognized that disabling and life-threatening injuries would happen again and again if these risk factors were not dealt with.

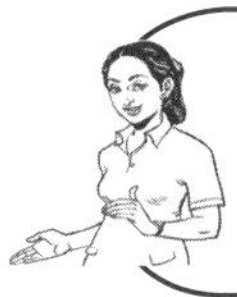

Take your group through the same process. It may be useful to consider the same questions Dula asked.

Risk factor identification

How to identify risk factors for injury

Dula asked her group to divide into smaller teams and walk through the village. She wanted them to look about them to identify factors that might cause injuries. She asked them to carefully observe the village layout, the environmental features, and the people of Dingly doing their daily tasks.

After the walk, Dula asked the group to give some examples of things they found that are known to cause the most common types of injury. Dula explained these are known as risk factors. She encouraged her group to think of risk factors in terms of the person injured, the energy source and the environment in which the injury happened. See, for example, Table 2.2.

Table 2.2 Risk factors: person, energy source, and environment

Type of risk factor	Risk factors
Injured person	• Alcohol consumption • Risky behaviour • Disease conditions
Energy source	• Unsafe products and equipment • Bath water too hot • Driving too quickly
Environment	• Unsafe motor vehicle design • Poverty • Large family size • Lack of safety standards, regulations, and laws • Unsafe road structure and lack of maintenance • Lack of safe cooking areas • Lack of safe play areas • Lack of safe national infrastructure and services

Dula explained that underlying risk factors, such as poverty, make it more likely that an injury could happen because there are many more risk factors. Risk factors that immediately contribute to the injury because they are close to where the injury (transfer of energy) took place, such as an open cooking fire, are called proximal risk factors.

Dula created another table, as shown in Table 2.3, by asking the group to arrange the same risk factors they had written in Table 2.2 according to whether they were underlying risk factors or proximal risk factors.

Table 2.3 Risk factors: underlying or proximal factors

Type of risk factor	*Risk factors*
Underlying factors	• Disease conditions • Unsafe motor vehicle design • Poverty • Large family size • Lack of supervision • Lack of safety standards, regulations, and laws • Unsafe road structure and lack of maintenance • Lack of safe national infrastructure and services
Proximal factors	• Alcohol consumption • Risky behaviour • Unsafe products and equipment • Bath water too hot • Driving too quickly • Lack of protective clothing and safety devices • Lack of safe cooking areas • Lack of safe play areas

Finally, the group created a further table that arranged the risk factors they had found in their village according to whether the factors related to the person and their family, or were features of the neighbourhood, or were structures and systems affecting the whole population. See Table 2.4.

Table 2.4 Risk factors: individual, neighbourhood and population level

Level of risk factor operation	*Risk factors*
Individual	• Alcohol consumption • Risky behaviour • Disease conditions • Bath water too hot • Driving too quickly • Large family size • Lack of supervision
Neighbourhood	• Unsafe products and equipment • Lack of protective clothing and safety devices • Unsafe road structure and lack of maintenance • Lack of safe play areas • Lack of safe cooking areas
Population	• Poverty • Unsafe motor vehicle design • Lack of safety standards, regulations, and laws • Lack of safe national infrastructure and services

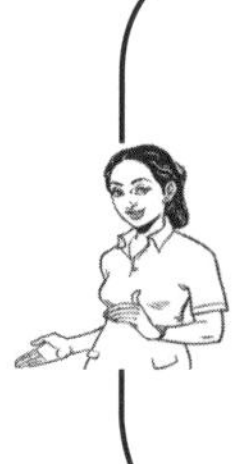

Dula's group came to understand that the transfer of energy causes an injury when a number of risk factors, both underlying and proximal at the individual, neighbourhood, and environmental levels, come together at the one time and place.

Take your group through the same process, using the same headings to help them see how the different levels of risk factors combine to cause an injury. Encourage them to see that by addressing the underlying risk factors, they will create an environment where there will be fewer proximal risk factors and therefore fewer injuries.

Intervention development and implementation

What is injury prevention?

Injury prevention is the process of creating and maintaining behaviour and environments that minimize the causes of injury in the community.

Prevention takes place in three phases: pre-event, event, and post-event. 'Pre-event' is the time before the injury happens. The 'event' is the point at which energy transfers to or from the body. The time after the injury is called 'post-event'. Each of these three phases provides an opportunity for prevention, as described in these examples.

- *Pre-event.* You can prevent young children on bikes getting head injuries from collisions with cars by stopping young children from riding bikes on busy streets.
- *Event.* You can also protect young children on bikes by making them wear bike helmets so that, even if they fall off, they are protected against head injuries.
- *Post-event.* If a child is injured, you can reduce the severity of the injury by immediately administering first aid and emergency care.

To be effective in preventing injury, death or disability, we must take action to reduce risk factors at the individual, neighbourhood, and environmental levels across all three phases.

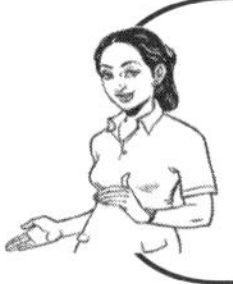

Encourage your group members to describe how injuries might be prevented in their communities during the pre-event, event, and post-event phases.

What can be done to prevent injury events?

Dula divided her group into three smaller teams. She named the first team 'Individual behavioural change', the second 'Neighbourhood environment modification', and the third 'Population regulation and enforcement'.

Each team discussed the risk factors they had written in their version of Table 2.4. They thought about actions that would prevent an injury event happening in their team's area.

Categories of pre-event interventions

To make a measurable difference in the number and severity of injuries, the most successful pre-event interventions have components from each of the three following categories. People change when multiple strategies make safe behaviour an easy and expected choice that benefits them. Interventions that simply give information do not work.

Individual behavioural change. If people understand what causes injuries and the benefits to them of preventing these events from happening, they are more likely to change their attitudes, beliefs, and behaviour. Providing information about the immediate and longer-term financial and emotional costs of injuries; media campaigns about common injuries; and public awareness campaigns about ways to avoid being injured can all contribute to changing behaviour and community expectations.

Neighbourhood environment modification. This approach works to remove risk factors from the environment (home, workplace, school, or road) and by making equipment (toys, machines, clothes) safer. This includes changing the engineering and design of the physical environment (e.g. creating smooth footpaths beside the road and moving cooking fires away from where toddlers play). The approach requires the people who create these physical environments (the builders of houses, the designers of roads, the mothers of small children) to change their behaviour.

Population regulation and enforcement. Enforcement of safety legislation is effective in reducing injury risk factors. The fear of a fine or penalty promotes safe behaviour across the whole community. Examples of population-level interventions include laws requiring the wearing of helmets on motorbikes, and regulations about safe building products and the use of toxic chemicals.

The GRIP Guide modules discuss the interventions that change behaviour, environments, and legislation for each injury type.

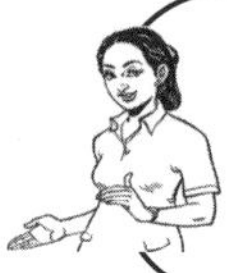

Ask your group members to work in three teams to discuss behavioural change, environment modification, and population regulation and enforcement activities that could be implemented in their community to prevent the injuries they discussed earlier.

Dula's group re-formed the small teams they were in when they walked through their village. She asked them to talk about what could be done to remove or reduce the impact of the risk factors they had seen. Each team wrote down the interventions they thought would work.

Dula reminded her group about the importance of understanding risk factors in terms of the person injured, the energy source or the environment; whether they were underlying or proximal risk factors; and also how they affected the individual and family, the neighbourhood, or the whole population.

The way the group thought about trying to solve the problems of injury was becoming increasingly sophisticated. The members had begun to realize they had many options and needed to work with a wider variety of people across the community.

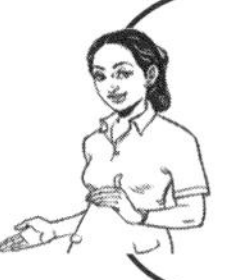

Ask your group members to repeat the exercise Dula's group did. If they are having difficulty, help each team by asking questions and providing the suggestions they may need to keep the ideas flowing.

Safety promotion

Safety promotion is another way to look at injury prevention. It encourages people to build on the underlying factors that protect a community from both unintentional and intentional injuries. Protective factors are strengthened when respect and trust are built through active participation and collaborative sharing of assets, strengths, and resources.

By promoting safety, the people of Dingly worked to establish a social and physical environment with fewer risk factors for injury and violence. To be effective and long-lasting, safety promotion required the whole community to be involved.

Community participation and collaboration. Dula asked her group members to form pairs and discuss what they understood by the words 'participation' and 'collaboration'. She asked them to think about the benefits of community participation and collaboration. When they came back to form one group, one of the members wrote the benefits on a large sheet of paper as each pair called their responses.

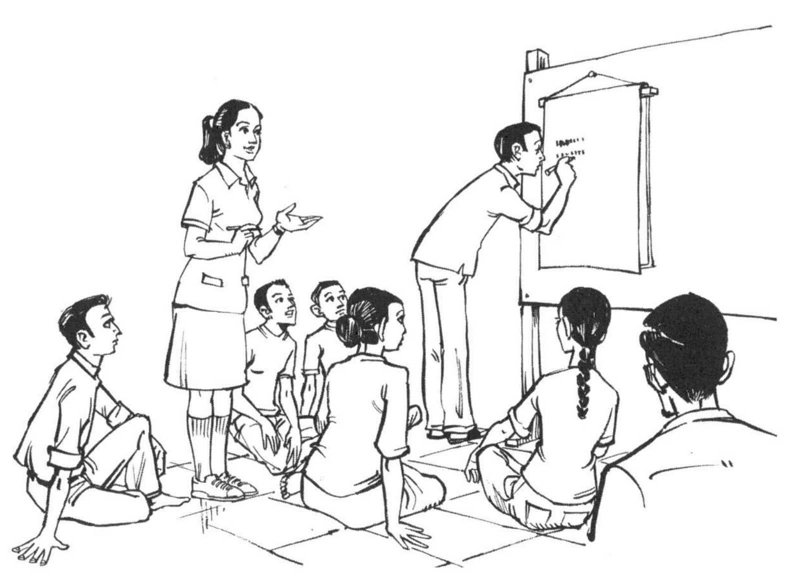

The group's list of the benefits of community participation and collaboration included:

- enables people to understand what is being done to make the community safer and why some things are seen as more urgent than others;
- builds community members' talents and confidence;
- enables skills and resources to be shared at no cost;
- gives community members a voice in developing the environments in which they live, work and play;
- encourages interventions to be in place longer and to protect more people;
- helps build relationships and understanding among community members with different interests and backgrounds;
- empowers the community to gain a greater understanding of issues that affect them all and to take positive action to improve their health and wellbeing;
- provides opportunities for community members and leaders to listen to the views of others and to express their own views more freely and openly;
- develops understanding, mutual respect, and acceptance of differences by creating opportunities for greater interaction and exchange of ideas.

Meaningful participation and collaboration can only take place when all those involved feel valued and respected as well as physically, emotionally, and culturally safe.

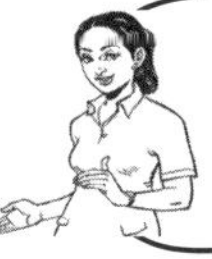

Community strengths, assets, and resources. Dula encouraged her group to think about Dingly's existing strengths and assets, and how people might be able to develop these to make the community stronger, safer, and more peaceful.

'Community strengths' could include the location of the village's natural resources, such as fertile soil and clean water; the variety of employment available; the number of people who can read and write; and the willingness of community members to live and work together.

An 'asset' or 'resource' is something that people have that is *valuable* to the community as a whole. While money is usually considered an asset, there are other assets that may be tangible and solid (such as a house) or more abstract (such as friendship).

Dula asked the group to again break into their smaller teams. Each team was asked to write down the strengths and assets they saw as belonging to Dingly. Table 2.5 lists the strengths and assets the group identified.

Table 2.5 Strengths and assets of Dingly's community

Individual	Neighbourhood	Population
Close family and friends	Fertile land	Government grants and funding for health, education, and transport
Friendly neighbours	Healthy and fertile farm animals	Accessible leaders who work with the community to improve the lives and futures of its members
Home-based care giving	Safe, clean water	Cultural traditions
Easy access to community resources and services	Healthy, productive crops and orchards	Temple/church/religion
Access to reliable information about current affairs	Shady vegetation and good pastures, community food gardens	Different types of businesses and employment
	Strong, well-built homes	Safe, well-maintained infrastructure
	Old people's homes/care services	Transport systems
	Crisis centres	Well-managed government services working to improve the community
	Social groups/organizations	Regulation and enforcement systems for alcohol consumption, occupational health and safety, and road design and construction
	Hospitals and primary health centres	
	Schools attended by all children	
	Police	

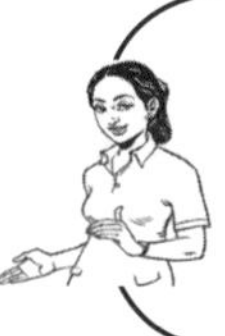

Explain the idea of a 'community asset' to your group. Ask them to break into smaller teams to list all the community assets they can think of in their community. Keep the list for the next exercise where they will think how they can use these community assets to develop their community into a safer place.

Community development. Dula's group agreed that 'development' meant 'making what is there better and available to more people'. They looked at the list of community assets and strengths they thought might be used to develop Dingly into a safer community.

Developing a safe and peaceful community requires the participation of many people from across the community (men, women, older people, younger people, unskilled workers, political leaders, professional people, business owners) and the collaboration of many agencies and organizations (non-government, government departments, church groups, international aid agencies).

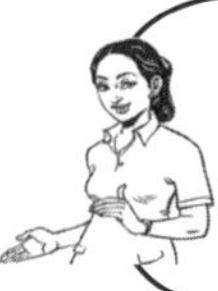

Divide your group into small teams, and ask each team to identify one community development intervention that uses existing population, neighbourhood, and individual assets to promote safety in the community.

Advocacy

Injury prevention and safety promotion depend on the ability of people to influence others through effective advocacy and leadership. Many of the structural and enforcement changes needed are beyond the control of health workers or individual members of the community. Advocacy is one way to expand your network of injury prevention allies to include those who are best placed to bring about real and lasting change.

ADVOCACY

Advocacy involves making a compelling case that will encourage others to act.

Increasing the knowledge and motivation of community and business leaders is an important step in injury prevention because many of the risk factors are at the neighbourhood and population levels.

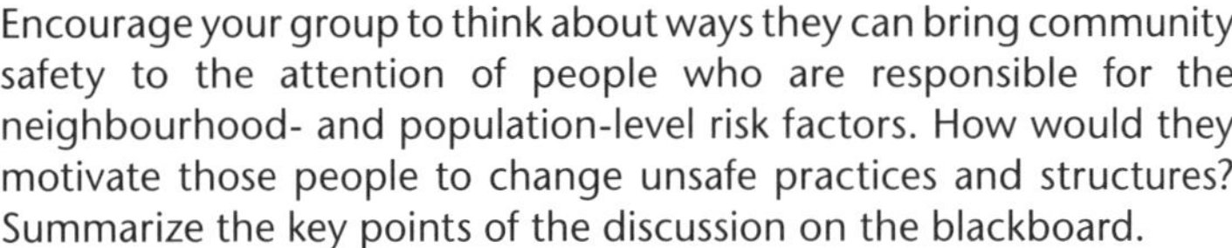

Encourage your group to think about ways they can bring community safety to the attention of people who are responsible for the neighbourhood- and population-level risk factors. How would they motivate those people to change unsafe practices and structures? Summarize the key points of the discussion on the blackboard.

Ask the group to focus on what needs to change and why. 'What must we do now? What can we do over the next three months? What do we need to do in the future?' Having a clear list of objectives and timeframes will enable the group to identify who they need to approach and what they want them to do.

What would be the group's most powerful argument to convince the decision-makers to take action? Finally, ask group members to discuss what other resources and community assets they might use to reinforce their argument.

Who should be involved? Dula's group understood that it was important that members were motivated to make real changes that would improve the health outcomes for the people of Dingly, rather than just discuss problems.

Dula asked the group to form pairs to talk about the people who have a potential role to play in preventing injury and promoting safety in Dingly. Following the discussion, the whole group came together and contributed to the list shown in Table 2.6.

Table 2.6 People with a role to play in preventing injuries

People	*Potential role*
Politicians	Make policy and legislation decisions that can remove or reduce exposure to injury risk factors at the individual, neighbourhood, and population levels Provide funding and resources to support the implementation of preventive policies and enforcement of protective legislation
Government officers	Implement policies and legislation designed to build and maintain safer communities
Non-profit organizations	Provide people and materials to support local injury prevention and safety promotion activities
Corporate sponsors	Provide people, money, and materials to support local injury prevention and safety promotion activities
International organizations	Provide expert advice and other resources to enable developing countries to prevent injuries and promote safety

(continued overleaf)

People	Potential role
Community leaders	Provide leadership and advocacy to bring about necessary changes in individual behaviour, modification in the neighbourhood environment, and enforcement of protective legislation across the community
Parents and family members	Create homes, gardens, and communities that are safe and free from the causes of injury Promote safe and peaceful communities free of violence and conflict
Workers and business owners	Establish safe work practices and ensure appropriate maintenance of equipment and storage of chemicals Follow safety precautions and use protective equipment
Print and radio media	Increase awareness across the community of the causes of injury Increase understanding of practical ways to prevent injury events

They were a little amazed at just how many people they could now see had a potential role to play in preventing injuries. Dula's group set out to invite people from the following groups to join the Dingly Injury Prevention Committee:

- people representing the diverse interests of the community (males, females, older people, younger people, parents);
- village head;
- public health staff of the village;
- representatives of community organizations and international agencies;
- the principal of the village school;
- representatives of local business owners and trade unions.

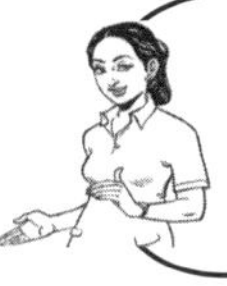

Ask your group to list the people who should be involved in injury prevention in your area. Does their list look like the one Dula's group came up with?

The group also realized that there were people who could provide important advice, guidance and advocacy, such as the local doctor and police officers, but whose work commitments might prevent them from being actively involved. The group was keen to draw on this advice and experience to help them bring about the changes needed to make a difference.

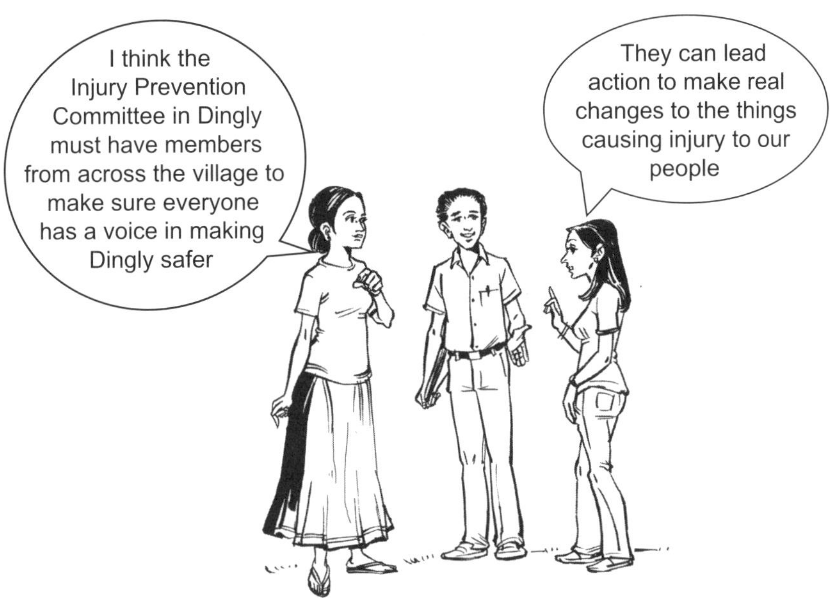

Dula's group identified the following people as potential advisers and powerful advocates:

- doctors at the village hospital;
- police officers;
- local council members;
- religious leaders;
- elected political leaders;
- local radio and print media.

Encourage the members of the group to think about the benefits there might be in involving people with different roles and responsibilities to work on preventing injuries. Support them to identify other potential members to provide advice and guide their injury prevention committee.

This may take some time to organize. There is no need to stop your group's progress; there is still a lot to learn by working through all chapters of this guide.

Progress monitoring

What information do you need?

Information is essential for influencing change in individual behaviour, environments, and regulations. It can help focus attention on specific types of injury or specific groups of people who most need protection.

Information is also necessary to monitor the success of interventions in removing or reducing risk factors. It will enable you to check that resources are being used where they will make the biggest difference.

Dula divided her group into teams of three or four members. She gave each team a piece of paper with a different category written on it:

- the nature and extent of the problem;
- priority areas for action;
- community assets and strengths;
- quality of interventions;
- ongoing evaluation and improvement of interventions;
- partner opportunities.

Dula asked each group to make a list of questions that could be asked about the category they were given. After a time, everyone came back into the large group to share their lists on the board, as shown below.

The nature and extent of the problem. Who is being injured? Where? When? How are the injuries occurring? How serious are the injuries? How many people have been injured? Under what circumstances are injuries occurring? Is the number of injuries changing over time?

Priority areas for action. Which injuries are most significant in terms of personal harms, and social and community costs? What interventions are currently available to reduce these costs? What is the evidence about whether these interventions work?

Community assets and strengths. What services and resources are available? Do services and businesses currently understand their role in preventing injury? Are injury prevention interventions working to protect all members of the population, especially those most at risk? Are community resources adequate to appropriately remove the injury problem?

Quality of interventions. Is the most reliable, up-to-date evidence used in the design and implementation of injury prevention and control interventions? Are the intended outcomes of the intervention clear? Are the strategies intended to support and reinforce change at individual, neighbourhood and population levels? Are all the people involved in interventions appropriately trained and supported? Is there a plan for continuous improvement, guided by appropriate ethical data collection?

Intervention evaluation. Is the intervention being implemented as planned? If not, what are the barriers to this happening? What can be done about the barriers? What benefits are being seen? How are the outcomes being defined and measured?

Partner opportunities. Are there other people who have an interest in the injury problem? What information do they have regarding the problem? What information do they need to motivate action? Can data and resources be shared to the advantage of all participating parties?

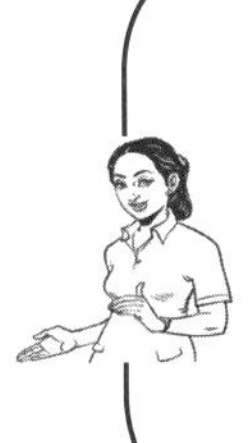

Support your group to think about the information they need to address the problem of injury in your community. Help them develop their list of important questions. Dula explained to her group that what they had developed was the framework for collecting information about injury in Dingly. Your group will follow this framework in later chapters of *The GRIP Guide* to assist them to collect the information they need to identify the problems in their village and to monitor how well they are doing with their efforts to make their village safer.

The prevention of injuries involves working with all the community to: count the number of injuries; identify the causes of the injuries; work out the best ways to prevent or remove the causes; and make sure strategies work together to remove as many causes as possible. When developing solutions, be aware of how the intervention is likely to be used, by whom, and in what environments. Interventions need to be acceptable to the values and practices of the target population.

The usefulness of your solutions is determined by how they are implemented in the community. A good outcome requires the community members to work together, supported by the social and political structures and institutions around them.

The GRIP Guide *helps you 'learn by doing', not 'do by copying'. Now is your chance to continue to help your community solve the problem of injury where you live.*

Part II

MODULE 1
BURNS

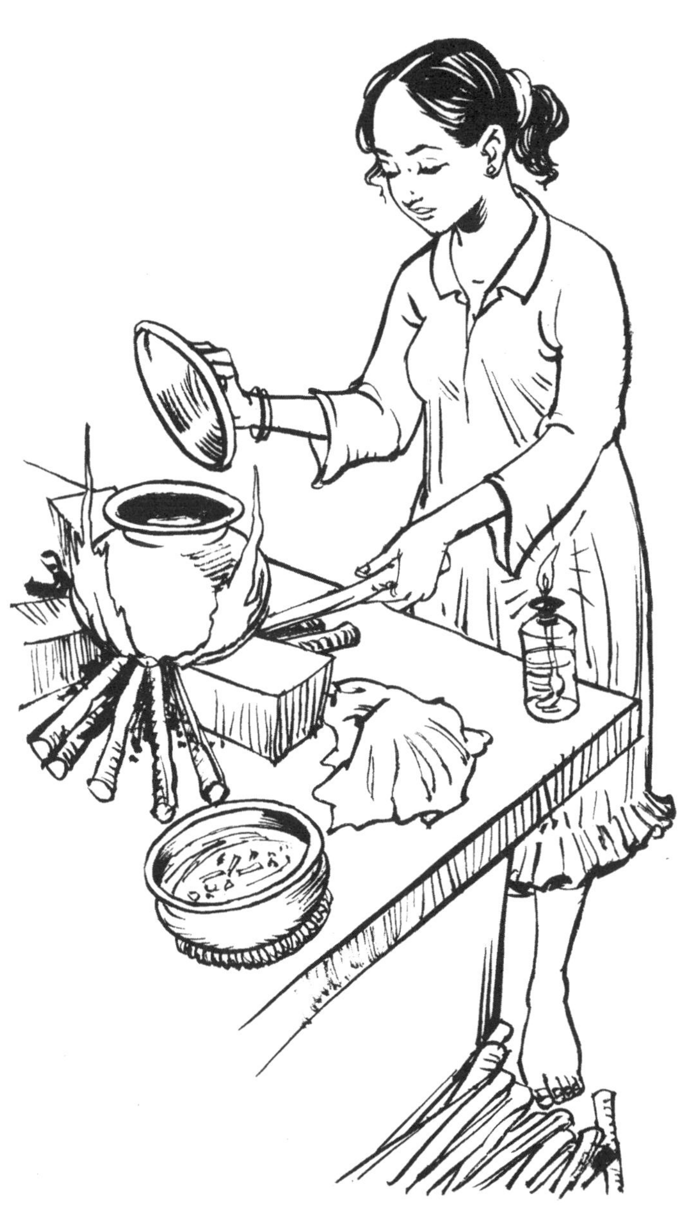

Burns occur when too much heat energy is transferred to the body. In any community there are personal, neighbourhood and population-level factors that increase the risk of people suffering a burn injury. You can help your community identify these factors by following the exercises in this chapter. Once risk factors for burn injuries have been identified, behavioural, environmental, and regulatory changes can be made to address the factors and improve the safety of the community. The chapter looks at how burns prevention interventions can be developed and implemented. When developing and implementing an intervention it is important to have clear aims for what you want to achieve within your specified timeframe. The chapter explains how to develop action plans to reduce burn injuries in your community and how to monitor the success of your plans.

Keywords: burn injury, cooking stoves, flames, fire, heat, injury prevention

Grasping the problem

Nihara, a 33-year-old mother of two young children, knocked over a kerosene oil lamp while cooking the evening meal. The overturned lamp spilled kerosene over her body and on to her nylon dress. The flame from the cooking fire quickly ignited the kerosene. Nihara suffered severe burns to most of her body and died at the local hospital two days later. The personal and financial costs to Nihara's family, and to the community as a whole, would be felt for years to come.

Dula knew this terrible event could have been prevented. She was keen to work with the Injury Prevention Committee and the people of Dingly to prevent similar tragedies. Dula realized that, to do this, they would need help to change people's behaviour; to modify the places where there was a greater risk of a burn injury happening; and to enforce the laws and regulations designed to protect people from injuries. They needed a collaborative approach, based on community knowledge and good local information.

As a first step, Dula invited the members of the Injury Prevention Committee to come together. The committee included people from different backgrounds and professions who had shown they wanted to find solutions to the problem of injuries in Dingly. Dula also invited others from the community, who had particular

http://dx.doi.org/10.3362/9781780448022.003

knowledge of the causes of burn injuries, to create a working group on the committee to address the problem of burn injuries in Dingly.

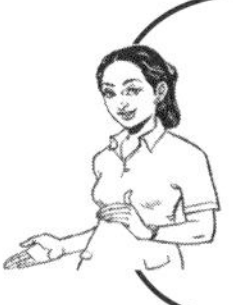

Encourage your Injury Prevention Committee to think about the people in their community who could help them prevent burn injuries. Invite the people on the list to the next meeting of the Injury Prevention Committee.

Dula started the first meeting of the working group by reminding the members that an injury is 'harm to the body caused by sudden transfer of too much or too little energy'. Burn injuries are caused by the transfer of too much heat from a source to a person.

To find a solution to the problem of burn injuries it is important that everyone in the working group has the same understanding of what the problem is. Start the discussions within your group by asking people to describe what they mean by a 'burn injury'. Using a 'talking stick' is a good way to make sure everyone is able to share their ideas and has an equal voice in the group.

You might help by explaining the definition of injury using ideas and examples from their everyday lives. Encourage people to talk about how their description fits with this definition.

When group members have agreed on a description that is meaningful to them, encourage them to think about the sources of heat energy in their community.

What are the sources of heat energy?

Dula's group shared their stories and ideas to create this list of sources of heat energy:

- fire;
- steam;
- hot objects;
- hot liquids;
- electricity;
- some chemicals;
- radioactive substances (radiation burns);
- two surfaces rubbing against one another (friction burns).

To start the group thinking about the physical, emotional, and financial costs of burn injuries, Dula had written three short case studies (stories) about injury events she had seen in her community field work. She was careful not to use real events involving real people as she did not want to cause further hurt to any group member by having them recall an injury or death of a friend or loved one.

Story 1

Piyal's clothing caught fire while playing in the kitchen near an open stove when he was four years old. He ran screaming out the door and around the garden until his mother was able to put the flames out. By that time he was severely burnt. Piyal's family feared the costs of his treatment and thought they could treat his injuries at home so he was not taken to the hospital until many days after he was burnt. By then the skin over his elbow and wrist had shrunk.

Now, at the age of 10, he has deep scars on his face, and his right arm and wrist are permanently locked in an awkward position. Piyal has not been allowed to enter the government school because he cannot hold a pencil. His parents worry about how their son will earn a living in the future.

Story 2

When Marina was five years old she accidentally tipped hot water over herself, scalding her face, right hand and chest. She suffered severe burns and permanent scarring. Marina is now 15 years old and extremely self-conscious about her appearance. She does not go out of her home unless fully covered and will not talk with strangers. Her father believes she will not find a husband and will be a burden to her family for the rest of her life.

Story 3

Kanthi is a 29-year-old pregnant mother of a one-year-old child. Kanthi was admitted to the emergency care unit with severe burns to her face, neck, chest, both arms and hands. She and her unborn baby died three days after admission to the hospital. Her drunken husband had knocked over the kerosene stove and the kitchen caught fire.

Dula divided the group members into smaller teams of three or four people and gave one case study to each group. She asked them to nominate a storyteller to read the case study and gave the teams about 15 minutes to talk about the possible immediate and future outcomes of the injury event described in the story. Dula asked each team to think about the outcomes for:

- the injured person;
- the family members;
- the community.

When everyone came back to form the large group, each storyteller presented a summary of their team's discussion. The following possible major outcomes of a burn injury were written on the flipchart.

Injured person

- pain and treatment over many months or years;
- permanent disability due to shortening and tightening of muscles and skin;
- scarring of the body and possible loss of fingers, hands and other body parts;
- impaired vision or permanent blindness if eyes were burnt;
- disrupted schooling and future education opportunities;
- loss of income;
- unemployment;
- depression, lack of self-esteem, and mental health problems;
- poor personal relationships and marriage prospects;
- death.

Family members

- costs of medication and transport to visit the family member in hospital;
- ongoing care of the patient;
- loss of family income;
- loss of the care and support previously given by the person to other family members.

Community

- costs of providing hospital treatment and ongoing rehabilitation services;
- loss of the injured person's contribution to the social life and future prosperity of Dingly.

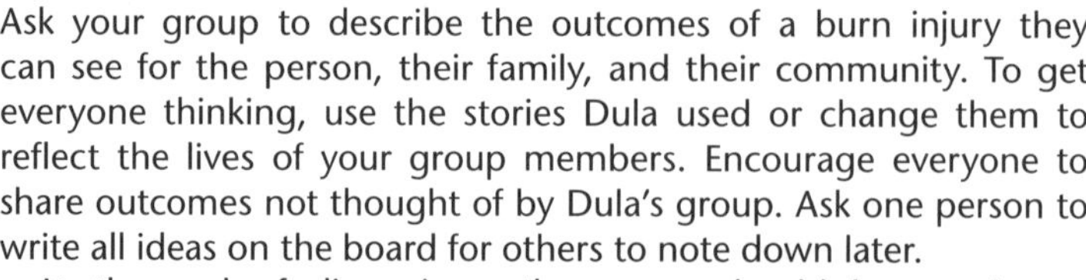

The nature and extent of the problem

Before they could think of effective ways to prevent burn injuries, the group needed to get an overall picture of the problem of burns in Dingly. They agreed to gather information to answer the following questions:

- Who is being injured?
- Where are the burn injuries occurring?
- When are the burn injuries occurring?
- How serious are the burn injuries?
- How many burn injuries have happened in the past year?
- What was happening when the person was injured?
- Are the numbers of burn injuries changing over time?
- Which burn injuries do the most harm in terms of direct costs to the community, and social and personal costs to the person and their loved ones?

Dula asked everyone to think about how they would get answers to these questions. One group member wrote the following suggestions from the group on the blackboard:

- police records;
- hospital or emergency department records;
- school records;
- workplace accident records;
- community surveys and event charts;
- discussions with community members, and industry and government representatives.

One person noted that some of this information was not easily available, pointing out they would not be allowed to go through police records. This prompted Dula to talk about gathering as much information as they could and finding answers from different sources to make sure the information was an accurate record. She stressed that information from just one source sometimes does not give a true picture.

Dula worked with her group to gather information from publicly available reports, newspapers, and other documents found in the library or from government offices.

She supported them to hold focus groups involving seven or eight people from a wide range of roles and experiences in the community. People from across the community (parents, older people, builders, community leaders, aid workers, school teachers, health workers, and government representatives) were asked the questions that the group had agreed were important in understanding the nature and extent of burn injuries in Dingly.

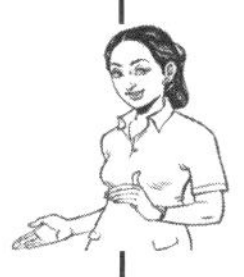

Encourage your group to discuss the answers they need to help them understand who is at risk, and how and where burn injuries are happening in their community. Help them to make a list of the questions they must ask to get the information they need to prevent these injuries. The group could choose to use Dula's questions or they might think of others that are important to their community.

Work with your group to list possible sources of information as they may not be used to doing something like this. Many universities, agencies, and government departments produce summary reports, so call on group members to write letters to, or visit, these agencies asking for information that will answer the questions about burn injuries in their community.

Ask members to talk with other community members and leaders from different ages and backgrounds to add their experiences to answer the group's questions.

Dula obtained the ethics approval and permission from relevant authorities before the group started collecting information from their community. Check with your local authority about what permissions you need.

Risk factor identification

Individual- and family-level risk factors for burns

Dula and her group discussed the information they had collected from the many sources and focus groups. Most people also had a story of a family member or a friend who had had a burn injury.

The information showed that most burn injuries in Dingly took place at home when people were cooking, or involved fuels for heating and lighting. It also told them that family members of all ages were at risk of a burn injury. To help everyone 'see' how these injuries could happen, one group member drew pictures on the flipchart of everyday scenes involving cooking, heating, and lighting.

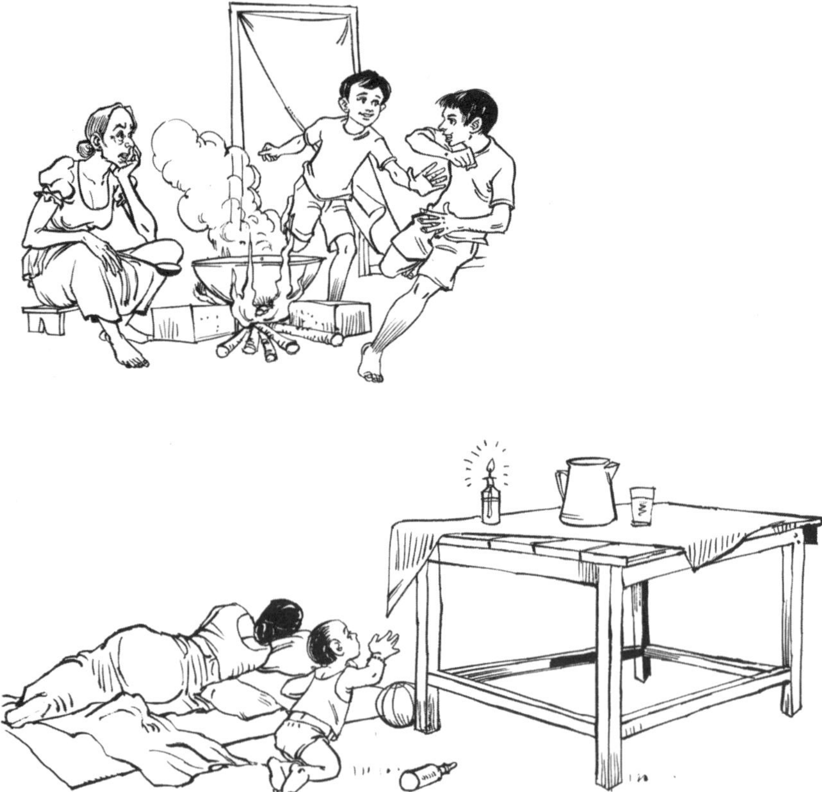

The group quickly identified risks in each picture. These included:

- Family members can accidentally fall into the fire.
- Embers can escape from the fire and ignite anything flammable.
- Pots can easily tip over.
- Hot pots are in reach of children.
- Children can pull out the burning firewood.
- Lamps can fall over, spreading burning oil and fire.
- Children can pull hot liquids or open flames onto themselves.

The group wanted to help family leaders understand that burn injuries were preventable and to change the things in their home that could cause burn injuries.

People in the village were still talking about the events leading to Nihara's injuries and so were willing to make changes to prevent the same thing happening to their family. Dula suggested that many villagers had told her they continued to do tasks in the home in the same way as their mothers and grandparents had because they had never thought about what might be changed to prevent burns and scalds. Dula told the group about action taken in other communities to give people the information they needed to make small changes to their home. The group decided to prepare a home burn risk assessment checklist using the information they had found at the library. The group persuaded an international aid organization to give them a small amount of funding each year so the checklist could be photocopied at the local council.

Before they gave out the checklist, they showed it to different community members to make sure it was useful and could be easily understood by everyone.

The group agreed that the list should be free and be made available in places used by most villagers, such as the local school, coffee shop, and markets.

Getting people to see the risks to their family was a good place to start but what was needed was action to change their behaviour and the risks in their home. Dula stressed that it would take many things working together for people to make these changes a part of their everyday lives. Any changes made would be short-lived if they were not made easy by having affordable safe ways to cook, heat water, and warm the home available to them.

What does the information the group has gathered tell them about burn injuries in their community? Discuss the risk factors for burns at the individual and family levels with your group.

What can they do to prevent or reduce these risk factors? Encourage your group to discuss the need for a home burn risk assessment checklist. Remind them that if they decide to use a checklist, they will need to make sure it is easily understood and helpful to all the people they want to use it. Work with your group to be clear on how the final checklist could be printed and made available to all family leaders over the coming years.

Neighbourhood-level risk factors for burns

Burn injuries in the workplace

The group's information showed that many people suffered preventable burn injuries in factories and workplaces. The group decided that the managers, maintenance officers, and workers were best placed to change the work practices and environments that put people at risk of an injury.

Dula and one group member met with managers, workers, and trade union representatives from a number of small and large workplaces to talk about the many outcomes and costs to them of injuries. They showed them the information about the number and type of workplace burn injuries in Dingly and explained that many of these injuries could be prevented.

Dula also reminded the business owners and managers that, under the law, they were responsible for the safety of the people working for them. She pointed out they could face charges and large fines if they could not show they had worked to protect their employees. She stressed that individual workers could do much to keep themselves and their workmates safe; however, they could only do this if they had the support of their managers.

The workplace representatives were keen to learn more about what they could do to prevent injuries. Dula showed them pictures of workplaces common in Dingly so they could talk together about the individual and environmental risks factors they could see in each workplace. She also encouraged them to talk about other risk factors they knew of from their own experiences working in Dingly and to suggest how these could be removed.

Workplace 1

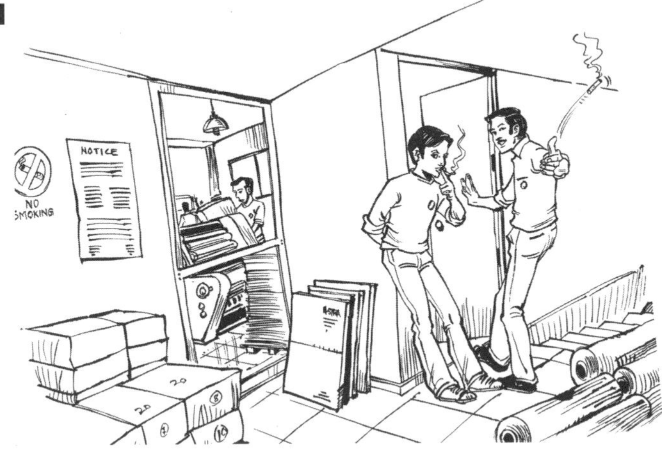

Workplace 2

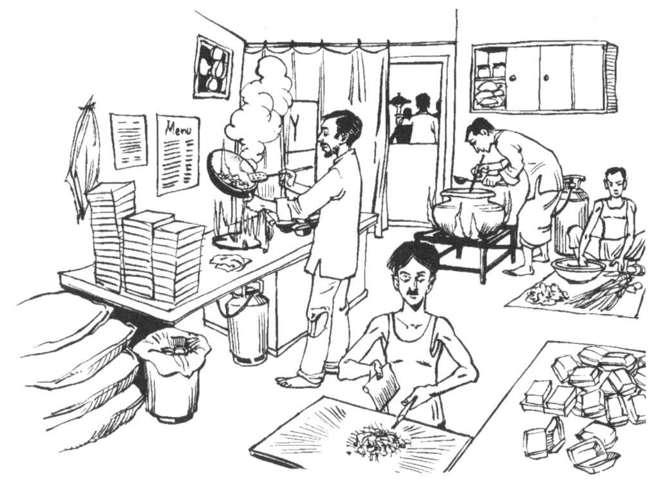

Workplace 3

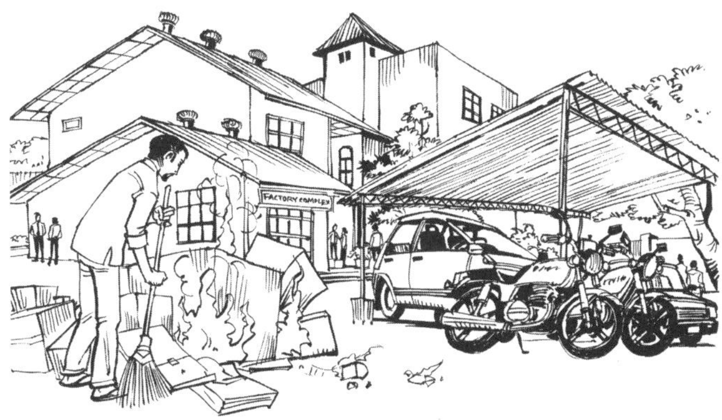

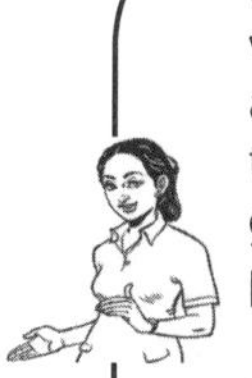

Does the information your group has gathered show that there are workplaces or jobs in your community where there is a high risk of a burn injury? Encourage the group to identify common activities that can lead to burn injuries in the workplace. To help people get started, use Dula's pictures if they are relevant to your area or pictures of workplaces common to the group's community.

Ask one person to write the suggested risk factors on the flipchart and encourage the group to discuss each one. What activities did people agree must be changed? Who is responsible for these activities?

Dula's group could see that many business owners, managers, and workers did not understand what they could do to prevent common burn injuries. They agreed that a simple list would help them look around their workplaces and factories for things known to increase the risk of injury. Dula asked managers, workers, and trade union representatives to help prepare a workplace burn risk assessment tool. The union agreed to print the assessment tool and make it available to all workplaces in Dingly for the next five years.

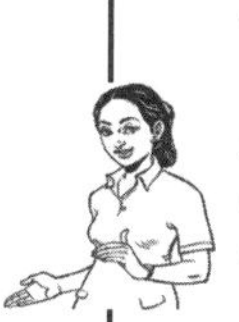

Your group members could use the same approach as Dula's group to involve managers and workers in taking action to reduce the number and severity of burn injuries in their community. Explain to your group that, to achieve lasting change, the people who are most affected by workplace injuries must be involved in finding the solutions. Changes that are forced on them will not last. If people cannot see a lasting benefit to themselves they will quickly revert to the old behaviour.

Encourage your group to discuss what might stand in the way of change in a workplace. Ask them to talk about what they can do to remove these barriers.

Discuss the workplace burn risk assessment tool developed by Dula's group.

Burns in local public places

The information gathered by the Injury Prevention Committee of Dingly showed that burn injuries often happened in public places, such as restaurants, halls, and shops. These places were often crowded, placing many people at risk.

Placing a large piece of paper at the front of the room, Dula asked her group to map the man-made structures and the location of activities in Dingly that increased the risk to the community of burn injuries. She asked people to form small teams to talk about the map while looking at the list of sources of heat energy they had identified earlier. The group could see the link between common community activities, the location of heat energy, and the history of burns to people in public places.

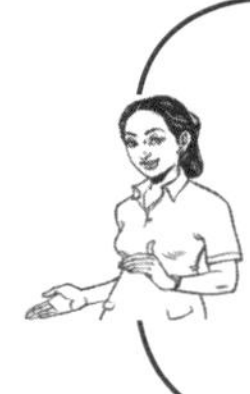

Ask your group to look at the list of heat sources they had identified earlier and to walk through the community to find risk factors for burns in public places. Arrange for your group to visit the local hospital and talk with hospital staff and patients about burn injuries. Did they get any information about burns in public places that they did not expect?

Population-level risk factors for burns

Dula and her group talked about the government systems and regulations that are designed to promote safe behaviour and to protect the whole community from injuries. It was agreed that the enforcement of the laws made people do things that helped prevent them and others from being badly injured or killed.

Dula's group found that the population of Dingly was not as well protected as it could be. They identified a number of major issues:

- There is no policy or law preventing the sale and use of unsafe stoves, lamps, and heating equipment.
- The existing workplace safety laws are not enforced.
- The punishments for breaking safety laws are not enforced.
- Inadequate attention is given to the prevention of burn injuries and the safety of workers.

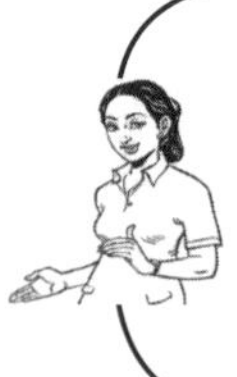

Intervention development and implementation

Setting aims for interventions

Dula's group thought about how much they had learnt over the previous weeks. They had increased their existing knowledge and experience in finding out the facts about burn injuries by working together. They had used the resources they had available to collect new information, and had learnt from talking with experts and from the books Dula had been reading. They now had a good understanding of actions taken in villages similar to Dingly to prevent burns.

Using all they had learnt, Dula and the group talked of the actions (interventions) that were needed to prevent burn injuries in Dingly.

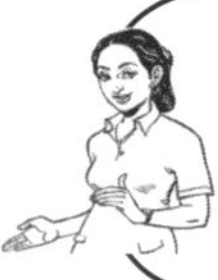

To make any real difference in the number and severity of burn injuries, they would need to agree on what they wanted to achieve, when it should be achieved by, and how they would know it had been achieved.

Dula asked them to describe what would be different after the interventions had been put in place as they planned. She explained that the final change they wanted would be their 'aim'. The proposed intervention should be sustainable, measurable, achievable, realistic, and time-specified (SMART).

Dula and the group brainstormed ideas about how they could make sure the benefits of their hard work would be seen in the future. After much discussion, the group decided that the aim of their intervention was: *to reduce the burns-related injuries and deaths in Dingly by 10 per cent each year for the next five years.*

To do this, they would need to involve the whole community in using the three strategies they now understood were critical to preventing injuries and promoting safety: behaviour change, environmental modification, and enforcement of rules.

Dula's group drafted the action plan for discussion with the whole village (see next page).

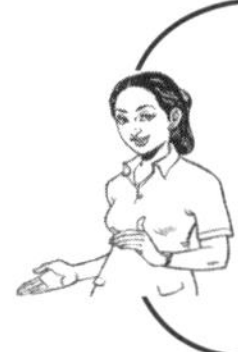

Encourage your group to be clear about what must change and how to continue the change into the future. Remind them to check that their strategies are doable; that the changes will become a part of everyday life; and that they can measure any difference in the number and severity of injuries over time.

Writing the plan made Dula's group realize there was much important work to do and that they would need many people working together to make the changes they had agreed were critically needed. At first the tasks seemed challenging, but Dula urged them to work on the activities agreed under one strategy before moving on the next.

Putting the interventions into practice

After a lot of discussion and sharing of ideas, Dula's group decided that the best way to get the community to give their ideas about the draft burn injury prevention action plan was to hold a free Community Information Forum. It was agreed that after the whole plan had been explained, the forum would focus on the activities listed under Strategy 1. They thought this would be the best way to:

- raise understanding that everyone in Dingly has a role to play in preventing burn injuries;
- gain approval of the draft action plan and gather support across the community to see activities implemented over the next five years;
- demonstrate safe, practical ways to make the home safer.

	THE DINGLY BURN INJURY PREVENTION ACTION PLAN
Our aim	To reduce burns-related injuries and deaths in Dingly by 10 per cent each year for the next five years
Strategy 1 *Activities*	Increase participation in injury prevention by people who are responsible for the causes of major burns-related injuries and deaths in Dingly • Work with mothers and grandmothers to increase supervision of children near cooking, heating, and lighting • Assist families to separate their cooking facilities from children's play areas with barrier protection • Support families to access and use safe cooking, lighting, and heating equipment • Encourage family members to wear tightly fitting, fire-resistant (cotton) clothing when cooking • Work with workplaces to set up proper storage of items that can catch fire easily • Support families, workplaces, and schools to develop and practise a fire escape plan
Strategy 2 *Activities*	Increase the number of collaborative projects across the community that are designed to reduce risk factors for burns-related injuries and deaths within the next five years • Work with property owners and builders to increase the use of fire-resistant materials when constructing houses, workplaces, and public buildings • Ensure appropriate storage of highly flammable materials in homes and workplaces • Establish 'no smoking' regulations throughout the community in areas of high fire risk • Work with manufacturers to increase the affordability and accessibility of safe lamps • Ensure all workplaces and public buildings have adequate fire escape exits, fire-fighting facilities, and fire escape plans
Strategy 3 *Activities*	Advocate to government and international aid groups to create and enforce injury prevention regulations across the community • Create opportunities for the community to get involved in advocating for structural and legislative changes to support individual and neighbourhood modifications • Convince governments, community leaders, and religious leaders to prohibit the sale and use of unsafe bottle lamps • Work with governments, community leaders, and religious leaders to ban the use of fireworks, except during authorized displays • Enforce laws against factory and workplace managers who do not obey safety standards in the workplace • Advocate for governments to ensure that the safety of the workers is considered when signing trade agreements with foreign investors

The group thought that once their intervention was fully accepted by the community, the activities under Strategies 2 and 3 could be more easily developed and put in place. The big advantage the group saw in this approach was that the early successes in the first stage would encourage the community to continue with the more challenging activities listed under Strategies 2 and 3.

Dula reminded the group about the importance of meetings being held in locations where all those present felt respected, valued, and emotionally and physically safe. She also pointed out that the forum should be held on a day and at a time that did not clash with religious, family, or work commitments of most villagers and community leaders.

The group suggested that Dula talk with the chief monk of the Dingly temple about holding the workshop in the temple hall as this was seen as a safe place of learning.

To show respect and to encourage the community leaders to see that they had a role in finding solutions to the problem of injury, the Injury Prevention Committee invited members of the village council to participate in the day. The council members agreed to provide lunch for those who attended. The doctor at the Dingly hospital agreed to talk about the burn injuries he treated. The presence of these community leaders was seen as helping in raising the importance of the forum in the eyes of the people of Dingly.

A number of days before the Community Information Forum, committee members posted notices in public places throughout the village and spoke on the community radio about where the free session was to be held, that lunch would be provided, and how the day would help the people of Dingly stay safe.

Many people who had suffered an injury urged their family, friends, and fellow workers to go. Dula and the group were delighted when most people of Dingly came to the forum.

Dula started off the day by describing the problem of burn injuries in Dingly. She used the case studies and information about local burns-related injuries to get people thinking about what caused the injuries. She spoke of the costs to the person, their family, and to the community. She told about the changes in behaviour, environments, and laws that have been shown to work in places just like Dingly.

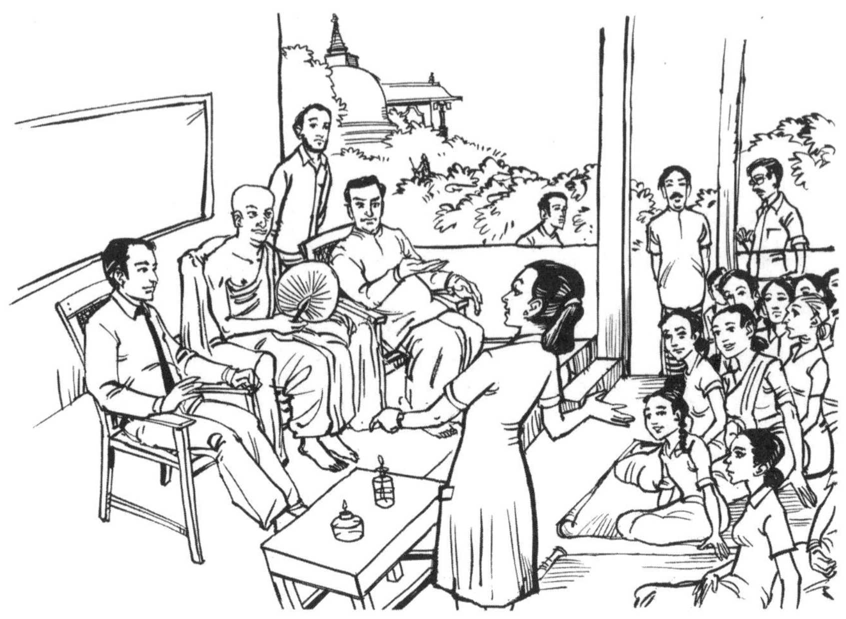

The local doctor described his experiences at Dingly hospital. He wanted people to understand that burn injuries happened to people of all ages, ethnic backgrounds, and incomes. He spoke about how and where the most common burns happened. Finally, he described some of the physical, emotional, and financial burdens that many of his patients and their families faced after a burn injury.

One of the members of the Injury Prevention Committee talked about the committee's work and read the draft burn injury prevention action plan. He explained that it was important to have a plan that would see activities build on each other and use the limited resources in Dingly to protect as many people as possible. The draft plan was approved by those present at the forum. The council members invited the committee to present the plan at the next council meeting and gave their support for the plan being put into action over the coming years.

Many people asked what they could do to help reduce the risks to themselves, their loved ones, and their community. Dula explained that there were many simple things that could be done now, such as making changes to how and where cooking was done. Dula had prepared a small demonstration of small changes that removed many of the main causes of burn injuries.

**Changing
where cooking
is done**

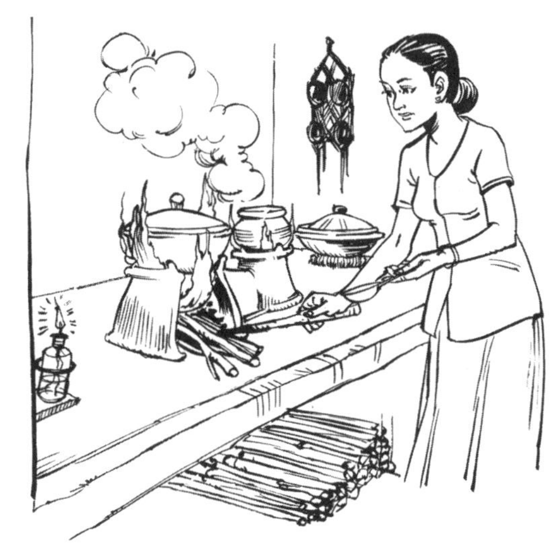

**Using lamps
that cannot spill
kerosene**

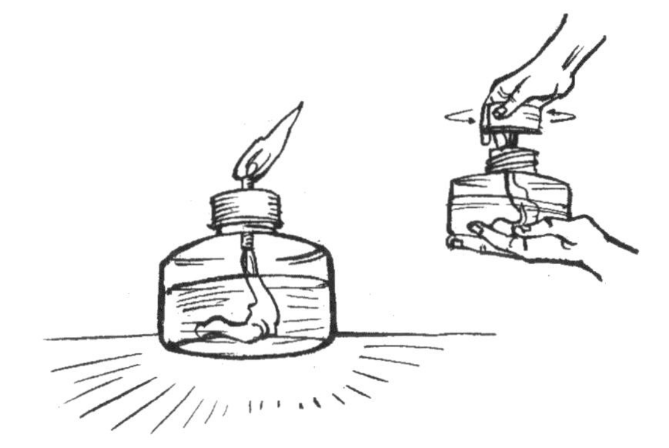

**Making safer
candle holders**

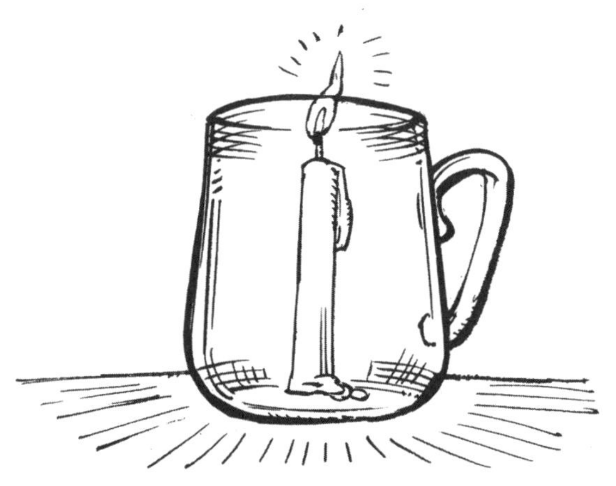

The doctor stressed that lives could be saved and burn injuries prevented if everyone knew what to do if there was a fire.

Making and practising a fire escape plan is a good way to help people get out uninjured if there is a fire in their home, school, or workplace. Dula went through what was in a fire escape plan and answered questions from those who were still unsure. She reminded the people at the information forum that the plan was only going to help if everyone in the home, classroom, or workplace knew about the plan and practised it every few months.

The information forum helped people from all parts of the community understand that injuries were preventable. They began to look about them for things they now knew were a risk for burn injuries. They could see that there was a lot they could do to help make themselves and their loved ones safer. Many people were keen to use the Dingly burn injury prevention action plan to make lasting changes to Dingly.

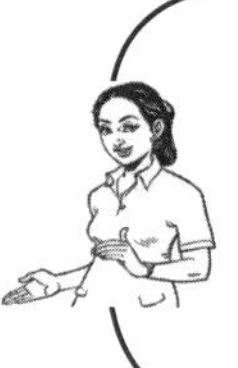

Ask your group to think about the assets and resources they have available to support them. Discuss how community members could best be encouraged to write and use a fire escape plan in their homes, schools, and workplaces. What other methods could they use to make burns prevention and fire safety a part of everyday life in their community?

Next steps

The people of Dingly started to build covered cooking stoves off the ground and out of reach of small children. As these stoves needed less firewood than open ground-level cooking stoves, they soon became popular.

After seeing Dula's demonstration and hearing the information about burn injuries in the home, most people also wanted to use safe lamps. The challenge was that the lamps were not widely available in Dingly and were too expensive for many families.

Dula talked with the manufacturers of safe lamps about training some villagers to make safe bottle lamps cheaply in Dingly. She told them about Nihara and others whose injuries could have been prevented if they had had a safe lamp. Dula pointed out that the manufacturers would not be losing income because the people of Dingly could not buy their lamps because of the cost. The manufacturers finally agreed to train three villagers, who did not have jobs, to make the lamps.

The Injury Prevention Committee obtained a loan from the local bank to start making safe lamps that most families could afford. As these lamps were cheaper and safer than the other lamps being used, most families bought them. The group started to sell the lamps to other villages and was able to continue making and selling safe lamps as a small-scale business.

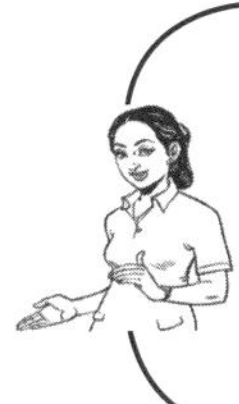

Ask your group to think about getting help from people outside their village to prevent burn injuries and to share ideas of small business ventures that improved the safety of their community while building its prosperity. Can your group suggest more low-cost changes that could be made to prevent burn injuries in their community? How are you going to introduce them into the community?

Dula's group was pleased with the community's response to the Community Information Forum. This first stage of the intervention had addressed many of the activities listed under Strategy 1 of their burn prevention action plan. Before the group began to put Strategies 2 and 3 into practice, they were keen to see (evaluate) how successful their implementation of Strategy 1 had been.

Progress monitoring

The success of the implementation of Strategy 1 was evaluated by collecting information to answer three questions:

1. Were the activities implemented according to the plan? (what was being done)
2. Were the desired changes in the community being achieved? (what had changed)
3. Were the number and severity of injuries decreasing? (the effect on common burn injuries)

To make it easier to answer these questions, the group developed an intervention monitoring worksheet. The worksheet was four pages – one page for each of the three main evaluation questions, and a final page that provided space to record which groups were being burnt (age, gender), where the burns occurred, and what activity was taking place at the time.

The information to answer Questions 1 and 2 on the worksheet was gathered by committee members every three months, while the doctors and staff of the local hospital and community health service agreed to collect the data needed to answer Question 3. The completed worksheets were collected and discussed at a meeting of the Injury Prevention Committee every three months, with changes made to the strategies to make them more effective as the needs of the community changed.

Dula and the Injury Prevention Committee agreed to hold a Community Information Forum each year to tell the community about the progress in changing behaviour, modifying environments, and enforcing protective legislation. Dula encouraged the community to celebrate the improvements that began to be seen in the number and severity of burn injuries.

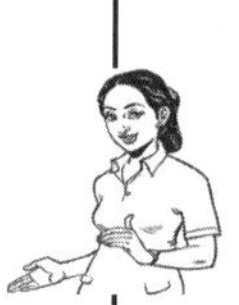

How will your group monitor the strategies they have decided to implement? Talk through the various options to decide how the information they need can be gathered.

Start their thinking by asking them the following questions: In what ways are you going to measure what is being done? How will you know what has changed? What has been the effect on burn injuries? How will the information be recorded? Who by? How will the information be used to improve the strategies? How long after the intervention has been finished will the information be collected? Where will the information be kept to help improve community interventions in the future?

Finding answers to these questions will help your group develop an intervention evaluation plan that will meet the information needs of their community.

Dula obtained the ethics approval and permission from the village leader and relevant authorities before the group started collecting information from their community. Check with your local authority about the permissions you need.

Dula used the community resources and assets to make safety promotion and injury prevention important to everyone living in Dingly. She supported local people to learn more, using local information sources, and guided them in making a plan of action designed to reduce the number and severity of burn injuries in Dingly. She involved the strong community leaders, the village priest, a council member, and the doctor. They were respected and had a big influence on the behaviour of many community members. Dula used many different ways to help make the people of Dingly aware of burn injuries and what they could do to prevent them.

MODULE 2
FALLS

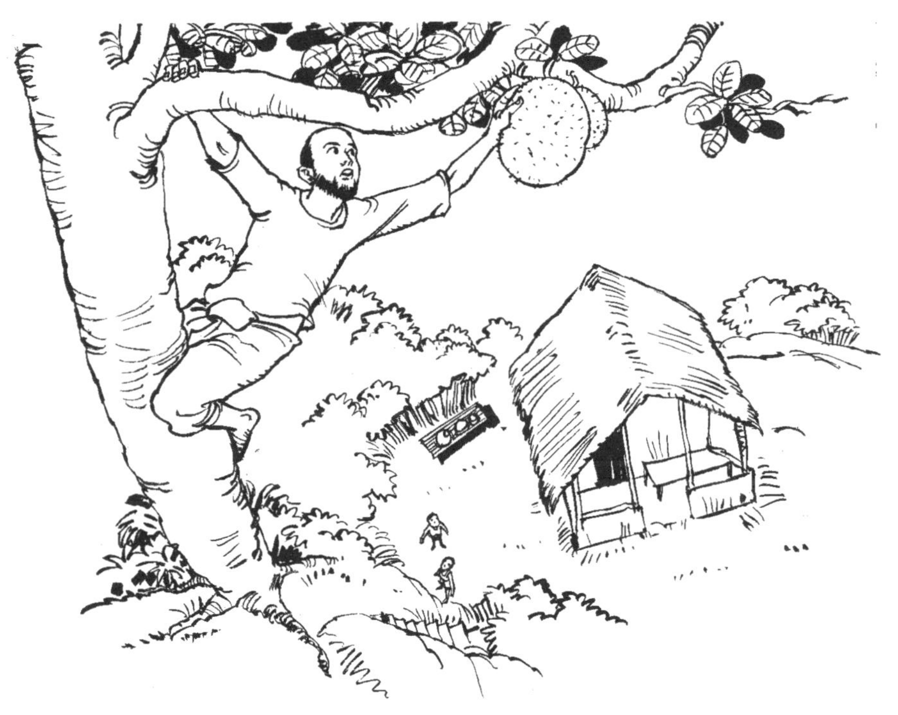

Falls are one of the most common types of injury in any community. They can occur in homes, workplaces, and the public environment throughout the neighbourhood. While some falls lead to only minor injury, other falls can lead to serious injuries and sometimes death, especially for older people or people who fall from a height. The risk factors for falls can be identified using a simple process described in this chapter. The chapter also describes how interventions to address these risk factors can be developed. A set of activities that encompass behavioural, environmental and regulatory interventions for the prevention of fall injuries is outlined.

Keywords: fall injury, fall from height, injury prevention, slips, trips

Grasping the problem

It had been raining continuously for three days in Dingly. Abdul, a 43-year-old manual labourer, was unable to work while the rain poured down so he could not buy food for his wife and four children. Abdul decided to climb a tree in his garden to collect some jackfruit, but missed his footing on the slippery branch and fell to the ground. His spine was permanently damaged. He is now unable to walk and is in constant pain. Abdul's 15-year-old daughter has had to leave school to look after her younger brother and sisters while their mother works to feed the family and cares for their father.

Abdul's injury was common in Dingly. Throughout the village Dula saw the physical, emotional, and financial costs of falls. These costs were often felt across the community for many years.

Work in other communities showed Dula that many falls could be prevented. The Dingly Injury Prevention Committee decided to invite people from all parts of the community to join with the committee to form a working group to address the problem of fall injury in Dingly.

http://dx.doi.org/10.3362/9781780448022.004

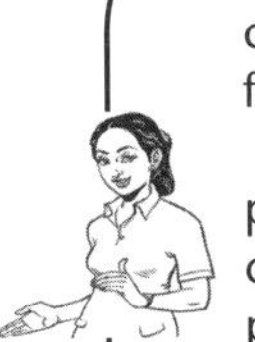

How would your group find out whether falls are a problem in your community? Ask one person to write all the suggestions on the flipchart where everyone can see.

Support your group to think about the people who have a role in preventing fall injuries. Is it more important for some people in the community to be involved than others? Why? What might motivate people to take action to prevent fall injuries?

Invite people who could have a role to play preventing falls to the next meeting of the Injury Prevention Committee. Ask them to be part of a working group to prevent fall injury in your community.

What is a fall injury?

Dula knew she needed a good understanding of what a fall injury was, who were most at risk of a fall injury, and the common causes of fall injuries in Dingly. She went to the local library, the local hospital, and her own injury prevention books to learn more about fall injuries. At the first meeting of the working group, she provided a definition of fall injury:

FALL INJURY

A fall injury occurs as a result of the energy transfer that happens when a person moves quickly and without control to the ground or floor, or other lower level.

To help the group understand this definition, Dula asked group members to think of what they mean by a fall and write their ideas on the blackboard. Dula discussed each response with the group. At the end of this discussion, the group worked out the common features of their different ideas.

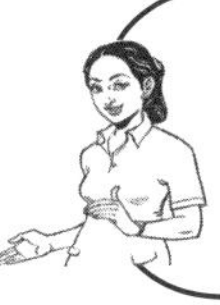

Encourage your group to talk about how their description fits with the definition found by Dula. Once the group members agree on a description that is meaningful to them, encourage them to think about the causes of fall injury in their community.

What can cause a fall?

Dula asked group members to think about all the ways they had described people falling. She handed out a set of pictures to the group and asked them to describe how each fall had happened.

Dula explained that the energy transfer that resulted in a fall injury depends on several factors, including:

- the height of the fall (the farther someone falls, the more severe the injuries are likely to be);
- the nature of the surface that the person falls onto;
- the part of the body that hits the surface;
- what protective gear is being used at the time of the fall.

Before your group can work to prevent fall injuries, it is important they understand what fall injuries are and what causes them. Draw on your reading to help the group understand what injury prevention researchers have learnt about the causes of fall injuries.

Encourage your group to share their ideas about how they can increase their understanding of fall injuries and their causes. Hearing many people sharing their stories of a fall injury can help make the size of the problem real to them. Ask group members to think about whether their experiences confirm the causes of falls found by researchers. If not, how was their experience different?

Ask your group to discuss each of the following pictures and consider the role of energy in fall injuries. Use a 'talking stick' to allow everyone to add their suggestions to the discussion. Ask one group member to write all suggestions on flipchart paper for all to see.

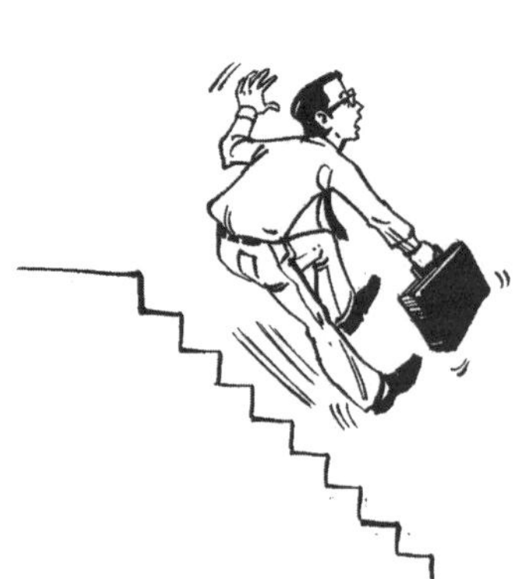

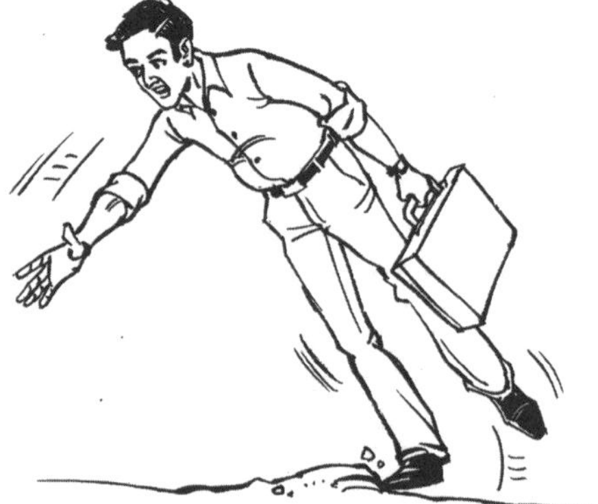

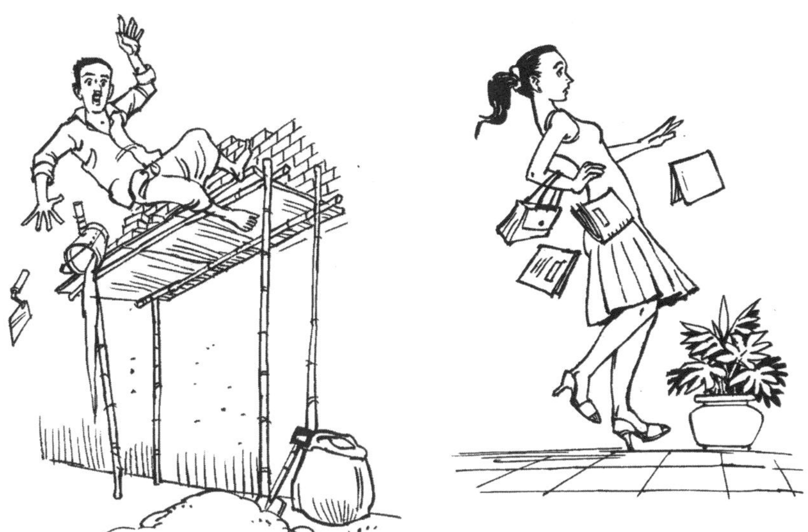

What are the outcomes of falls?

Dula gave each group member a piece of paper and asked them to write an outcome of a fall and then form pairs to discuss their ideas. After about 10 minutes, Dula called her group back together to share the key things each pair had talked about. There were many stories and the group agreed the outcomes of the falls not only affected the life of the injured person but also the lives of their family members and the community as a whole.

Injured person

- fractures (breaking of bones);
- dislocations (displacement of joints);
- abrasions and lacerations;
- cuts;
- bruising;
- permanent disability such as loss of sight, hearing or the ability to speak, loss of mobility;
- hospitalization for short or long periods of time;
- missed school or work;
- lost future expectations for both the injured person and their family and friends;
- death.

Family members

- loss of the care and support given by the injured person;
- cost of medication and treatment;
- ongoing care of the injured person;
- reduced family income.

Community

- cost of providing hospital treatment and rehabilitation services;
- loss of a community member able to help build the future of the village.

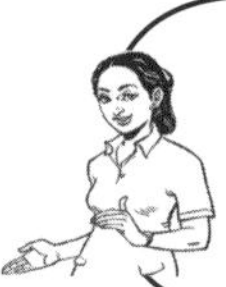

Ask your group to add to the outcomes identified by Dula's group. It is important that your group understands the impact a fall can have on their community. This will help them think about how best to motivate others to take preventive action.

The nature and extent of the problem

Dula was keen for the group to know more about the most common falls in Dingly. The group agreed that they needed answers to the following questions:

- Who is being injured?
- Where are the fall injuries occurring?
- When are the fall injuries happening?
- How serious are the fall injuries?
- How many fall injuries have happened in the past year?
- What was happening when the person was injured?
- Are the numbers of fall injuries changing over time?
- Which injuries are most significant in terms of direct costs, and social and personal harms?

Dula worked with her group to gather information about fall injuries from the local hospital and emergency department records, workplace accident records, community surveys, and from discussions with people from across the village.

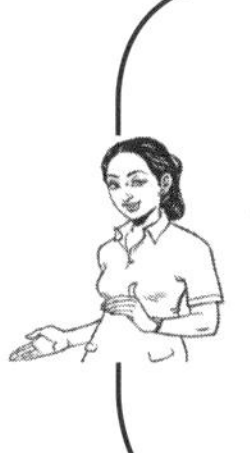

Each community is different, with different resources and access to information. Knowing when, where, and to whom fall injuries are happening will help your group use the right community resources to prevent fall injuries. Encourage your group to work together to decide how they can find answers to the above questions, even in isolated and poorer communities. Remember to make sure everyone has a chance to ask questions and to join in the discussions to find solutions.

Dula asked everyone to look carefully at the information they had gathered and challenged them with the question: 'Who is most often being injured by a fall in Dingly?' The group quickly agreed that the information showed that the answer was older people, workers, and children.

Risk factor identification

Individual- and family-level risk factors for falls

One person asked why older people, workers, and children were more at risk of a fall injury than others. Dula invited the whole group to call out their answers to this question. One group member wrote the suggestions on the board. The group saw that there were factors at the individual, environmental, and community levels that all increased the risk of a person falling.

Individual- and family-level risk factors for injuries due to falls include:

- lack of knowledge about ways to protect against falling in the home, workplace or street;
- older people not taking their proper medication or nourishment, causing low blood pressure and dizziness;
- older people lacking sufficient strength and balance to avoid tripping or slipping;
- wearing non-fitting footwear, or footwear with poor tread on the sole;
- not wearing protective clothing and harnesses at work;
- lack of supervision of children and older people to help them avoid hazards.

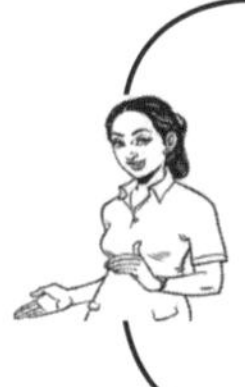

> Encourage each person to share their personal experiences and the things they believe led to their fall. You might help them by asking what were they doing (and not doing) to keep themselves safe, where they were, and what the surrounding environment looked like. Your group may think of factors to add to Dula's list. This will make a good base to use later when they start to plan action.

Environmental or neighbourhood-level risk factors for falls

By looking at the information they had gathered, the group saw that most injuries happened in three main places: the playground, the home, and the farm or other workplace.

The group formed three small teams. These teams set off to visit school playgrounds; a selection of homes; or a number of farms, workplaces, and construction sites. It was important to visit a number of similar places, not just one, to ensure that the things they saw were common to many sites rather than found in just one.

Dula asked each team to list as many risk factors for fall injuries as they could see. The teams talked with the people they met to learn more about the location and the common activities in that place. They noted the things that could cause someone to be injured by a fall. Their visits encouraged people in Dingly to think more deeply about their own risk of falling and to start asking what they could do to reduce this risk.

Each group presented their findings to the larger group and listed them on the flipchart.

Risk factors in the playground

- no protective surfacing under or around the play equipment;
- some play equipment too high above the ground;
- no protective guardrails or safety barriers on elevated platforms, bridges, walkways, and ramps;
- some parts of the play equipment not properly fitted or jutting out into play areas.

Risk factors in the home

- children playing in unprotected areas such as on roofs, balconies, and stairways;

- lack of maintenance leading to loose floorboards or weak guardrails on windows and balconies;
- liquids spilt on the floors or walkways;
- walkways and floors covered with clutter, such as rubbish, tools, or mats;
- dark, uneven walkways and poorly lit stairs;
- lack of handrails on stairs;
- no guards on windows;
- no non-slip mats in washing and bathing areas;
- poor maintenance of the garden leading to exposed tree roots and fallen branches.

Risk factors at farms, workplaces, and construction sites

- wet surfaces;
- obstructed walkways;
- untidy, cluttered floors;
- uneven, poorly maintained floor surfaces;
- changes in floor level (steps, stairs, slopes);
- workers carrying loads on stairs;
- inappropriate footwear;
- inappropriate structures, such as chairs, used to reach heights;
- inappropriate or unsafe ladders;
- inappropriate use of elevated work platforms;
- unprotected raised platforms;
- missing or damaged grates or covers of floor openings;
- no safety harness or equipment used when climbing trees and other high structures;
- coir ropes that connect tops of the trees used to go from one tree to another;
- no guardrails or safety barriers on raised loading platforms;
- wells and sewage pits left uncovered.

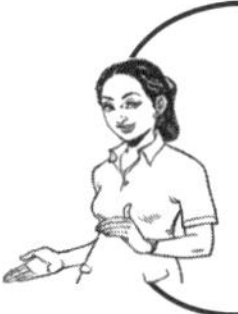

A lot can be learnt by visiting the places in the community where fall injuries happen. Encourage your group to discuss how they would go about arranging field visits to gather the information they need to fully understand the risk factors for falls in their community.

Population-level (structural) risk factors for falls

The group talked about structural risk factors that increased the risk of fall injuries in Dingly. One group member wrote their thoughts on a flipchart page.

- There are no policies, regulations or laws relating to the safety of houses, factories, and construction sites.
- The level of poverty in the village meant that safe options were often not available.
- The lack of monitoring of medication and the cost meant that older people often shared their medication with others or did not take the correct dose ordered by the doctor.

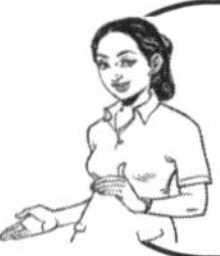

Ask your group to think about the population-level risk factors for fall injuries in their community. What systems need to be put in place to ensure the local environment is safe for all community members?

Intervention development and implementation

Dula knew there was good evidence from other communities that fall injuries were preventable and that a community could do things to address the problem. She was keen for her group to hear about the great work done in other areas in reducing a major risk for fall injuries. Dula told her group about the Children Can't Fly programme.

'Forty years ago, the healthcare staff of Jacobi Hospital in New York noticed that children were being admitted after falling from windows. Some of them died and some had long-term disabilities resulting from broken arms or legs, and brain injuries.

'The New York City Department of Health started a health education programme, called Children Can't Fly, which aimed to stop children falling from windows. First, they wrote a plan outlining strategies they had designed to make the safest option the easiest one for people to choose. They knew that telling people to change would not work unless it was made as easy as possible for people of all incomes to put their new knowledge into action. Some of the ways they did this were as follows.

- New parents were visited to talk about the risks to their young ones caused by open, unprotected windows and balconies.

- Free leaflets were distributed, telling people what they could do to help keep their children safe from fall injuries. These leaflets had lots of pictures to make it easy for people with poor reading skills to get the information they needed.
- Free television, radio, public service spot announcements, and news stories delivered simple safety messages.
- A voluntary system reported all falls from windows and arranged follow-up home visits by trained health workers to help the parents prevent this happening again.
- Free, easily installed window guards were provided to families with preschool-aged children.
- A new law required that window guards be installed in all high-rise buildings.

'Five years after starting the programme, falls from windows had halved.'

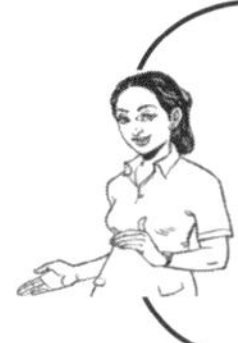

Telling stories about the success of others can motivate people and provide examples of what can be useful when planning fall injury prevention strategies. Share the Children Can't Fly story with your group and encourage them to discuss what they could do in their community to prevent injuries from falls.

Setting aims for interventions

The Dingly group agreed that if their work was a success, there would be much less harm from falls. This enabled them to write the aim of their intervention as: *to reduce fall-related injuries and deaths in Dingly by 10 per cent each year for the next five years.*

Under the aim, they wrote down a series of activities that would address the individual- and family-, neighbourhood-, and population-level risk factors. These activities involved each of the three strategies they knew were critical to prevent injuries and promote safety: behaviour change, environmental modification, and enforcement of rules.

Dula wrote two questions on the board to help the group focus its thinking about the steps required to achieve their aim:

- What is currently available to prevent fall injury in Dingly?
- How do we know which preventions will work?

Dula's group drafted the action plan for discussion with the whole village (see next page).

<table>
<tr><td colspan="2" align="center">THE DINGLY FALL INJURY PREVENTION ACTION PLAN</td></tr>
<tr><td>Our aim</td><td>To reduce fall-related injuries and deaths in Dingly by 10 per cent each year for the next five years</td></tr>
<tr>
<td>Strategy 1

Activities</td>
<td>Increase participation in injury prevention by people who are most at risk of fall-related injuries in Dingly
<ul>
<li>Encourage older people to wear appropriate, properly fitting, non-slip footwear</li>
<li>Encourage older people to have their medications reviewed by a professional to make sure they are not increasing the risk of falling</li>
<li>Encourage older people to do regular exercise and physical activity that improves their strength and balance</li>
<li>Work with mothers and grandmothers to increase supervision of children and older people in places where they could fall</li>
<li>Raise awareness about the steps people can take to reduce the risk of falling in their daily life, such as wearing harnesses when climbing, holding on to rails, removing loose mats and avoiding slippery places</li>
</ul>
</td>
</tr>
<tr>
<td>Strategy 2

Activities</td>
<td>Increase the number of collaborative projects across the community designed to reduce risk factors for fall-related injuries and deaths
<ul>
<li>Work with schools and local councils to address the risks for falls in playgrounds by:
<ul>
<li>building protective surfacing under or around the play equipment</li>
<li>keeping play equipment at a safe height above the ground</li>
<li>ensuring there are protective guardrails or safety barriers on elevated platforms, bridges, walkways, and ramps</li>
<li>ensuring all surfaces are smooth and properly fitted, and do not jut out into play areas</li>
</ul>
</li>
<li>Work with families to address the risks for fall injuries in the home by:
<ul>
<li>installing barriers to prevent children playing on roofs, balconies, and stairways</li>
<li>making sure verandas and balconies have a proper guardrail of the right height</li>
<li>encouraging proper maintenance of houses to minimize loose floorboards and weak guardrails on windows and balconies</li>
<li>cleaning up liquid spills on the floors and walkways</li>
<li>removing rubbish, tools, and toys from walkways and floors</li>
<li>installing good lighting for walkways and stairs</li>
<li>installing handrails on all stairs</li>
<li>building guards on windows where children could climb out and fall</li>
<li>placing non-slip mats in washing and bathing areas</li>
<li>properly maintaining gardens to reduce hazards</li>
</ul>
</li>
</ul>
</td>
</tr>
</table>

<table>
<tr><td colspan="2">THE DINGLY FALL INJURY PREVENTION ACTION PLAN
Our aim   To reduce fall-related injuries and deaths in Dingly by 10 per cent each year for the next five years</td></tr>
<tr><td></td><td>

- Work with managers and workers to address the risks for fall injuries on farms, workplaces, and construction sites by:
  - keeping surfaces dry
  - clearing walkways and tidying floor areas
  - maintaining even floor surfaces
  - ensuring workers have appropriate footwear
  - enforcing standards for lifting and carrying of material
  - ensuring safe practices for climbing ladders and platforms
  - installing guardrails around all platforms when working from height
  - wearing safety harnesses at all times when working at height
  - ensuring wells and pits are covered

</td></tr>
<tr><td>Strategy 3

Activities</td><td>

Advocate to government and international aid groups to create and enforce injury prevention regulations across the community

- Create opportunities for the community to get involved in advocating for structural and legislative changes to support individual and neighbourhood modifications
- Work with governments and professional groups to develop policies, regulations or laws relating to the safety of houses, factories, and construction sites
- Encourage authorities to enforce laws against factory and workplace managers who do not obey safety standards in the workplace
- Work with professional groups (such as doctors and pharmacists) to encourage routine monitoring of medication taken by older people and to discourage them sharing their medication with other people
- Increase government awareness of the need to build fall prevention into their policies

</td></tr>
</table>

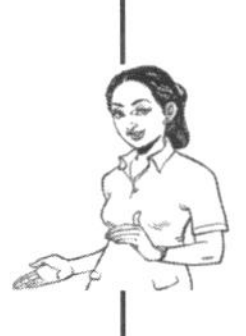

Dula and her group first determined the broad aim of their proposed intervention and outlined what they hoped to achieve. Then they identified behavioural change, environment modification, and regulation as the strategies for achieving this aim. Work with your group to set aims for your interventions to reduce the injuries caused by falls in your area.

Encourage your group to be clear about what they must do to make change not only happen now but continue into the future. Remind them to check their strategies are sustainable, measurable, achievable, realistic, and time-specified (SMART).

Putting the interventions into practice

One person in Dula's group pointed out that there were limited resources to tackle the many risk factors for injury in Dingly. He asked how the community could make a difference when most injuries happened in such diverse places as playgrounds, farms, and workplaces.

Dula encouraged them to see that one way to tackle such a big task is to make a start on fixing things you are able to change reasonably easily and keep working on the more difficult issues over time. If the community sees they are making a difference, they will be motivated to keep going with the challenges ahead.

To make a start, the working group went around Dingly to speak to many people about the injuries they, or others, had as a result of a fall. They talked to farm owners, community leaders, older people, healthcare providers, and the school principal about the physical, social, and financial costs of many fall injuries. The group talked about how researchers and other communities similar to Dingly had been able to show that falls could often be prevented by making changes to people's behaviour and the environments in which falls most often happened.

The group was able to deliver a strong message about the need for action and soon had a number of people eager to get to work on making their homes, workplaces, and village safer.

Dula and the group looked at the assets the community had available that they could use to implement the action plan. They wrote a list of the people who could be interested in being involved in the proposed activities. This included:

- education managers;
- retired people in the village;
- the public health team of the village;
- school teachers;
- parents;
- factory owners and managers;
- leaders of trade unions;
- the business community.

Dula and the group went to all the settings in Dingly where fall injuries were a problem. They visited the child immunization clinics and antenatal clinics of the area to talk about prevention of falls among children. They arranged for practical advice about safety to be given to mothers of young children.

They visited the gatherings of older people in Dingly and talked to them about their risks of fall injuries and how to prevent them. They stressed the importance of:

- changing their homes to protect people from slipping and tripping;
- eating a balanced diet;
- taking only prescribed medication;
- wearing properly fitting footwear;
- having frequent medical check-ups;
- attending strength and balance training classes if they were not getting regular exercise.

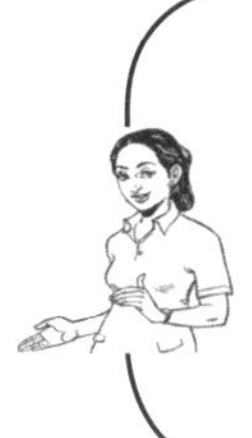

Dula and the group could not visit all the houses of Dingly, so they selected the places where groups of the most-at-risk people often gathered in the community. They delivered different messages about falls prevention to raise awareness of common causes of injury to each different group. Think of such group gatherings in your community and outline the messages you could give to meet the information needs of each of these groups.

Initially, it was difficult for Dula to get permission from employers to conduct a workshop about preventing falls in the workplace. She managed to convince one factory manager of the advantages of preventing injuries and improving the safety of the workers. This factory manager allowed Dula to conduct a workshop on the prevention of falls at the factory. Both managers and workers participated in this workshop.

At the beginning of the workshop, Dula briefly talked about the injuries that can occur from falls. Then she explained the advantages of preventing these injuries for both employers and employees. She stressed the money that could be saved by the factory owner by having a safe workplace. They discussed their experiences of falls and fall injuries in the workplace and the resources they could use to prevent fall injuries. The workshop group members drafted a workplace falls prevention plan for use by employers and workers to prevent falls in the workplace. As both employers and employees participated in the workshop, and were involved in the preparation of work plan, they felt they were responsible for its implementation.

After the successful workshop in this factory, other factory managers heard about it and invited Dula to conduct workshops at their factories to help them prevent falls among their employees.

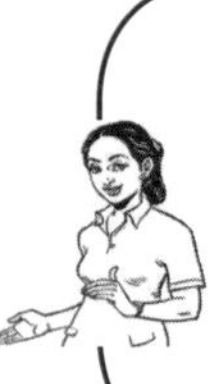

A workshop is one of the most effective ways to form a plan for action. Could you conduct such a workshop in your area? It is important to have a facilitator to keep the discussion heading in the right direction and encourage participation of all the members. Finish the workshop with a decision about what you plan to do and when you are going to do it. Could your group develop a workplace falls prevention plan to suit workplaces in your area?

Dula's group also worked on improving falls safety in public places. For example, they lobbied policy makers to set up rules and guidelines to prevent injuries due to falls when building houses and factories. They worked with the local council to gain funds to install handrails in public places in Dingly.

The group next decided to make playgrounds in Dingly safer. Based on her reading and discussions with school leaders, Dula worked out guidelines for building safer playgrounds. The fathers of Dingly used locally available building materials to bring the village playground up to safety standards. The village youth club agreed to maintain the playground to the recommended safety standards into the future.

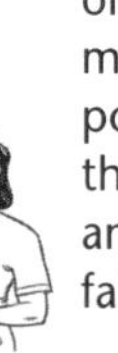

As a responsible community health worker, Dula provided information on playground safety guidelines. She encouraged the community members to use locally available low-cost materials as much as possible. By involving the youth club in maintaining the playground, the group ensured the good work would continue. Could you plan and carry out some activities to modify your community to prevent fall injuries and improve the safety of your community?

Community workers can influence policy makers to establish new rules and guidelines that prevent fall injuries in our communities. Dula and the group lobbied the council members to achieve this task. What strategies would you use to advocate on behalf of your community to work towards change in government policy?

Dula's group was encouraged by the community's response to their initial efforts and planned to keep their playground falls prevention intervention going for five years. Even in the early stages they were keen to evaluate how successful their efforts had been and wanted to learn what they should do next. So they undertook to monitor progress against their agreed Falls Prevention Plan.

Progress monitoring

To help the group track whether they had made a difference so far, they developed an intervention monitoring worksheet that they could complete.

The worksheet was four pages long. On the first page, they recorded information that would tell them whether the activities were implemented according to their plan. On the second page, they noted whether the desired changes in the community had been achieved and gathered evidence to support these findings. On the third page, they recorded information about whether the number and severity of injuries was decreasing. A final page provided space for recording who was injured (age, gender), where the falls occurred, and what activities were taking place at the time.

These questions were useful to monitor the effect of the strategies and to provide additional information that could be used to adapt the strategies as the needs of the community changed.

The doctors and staff of the local hospital and community health service agreed to collect information on the intervention monitoring worksheet. The information was collected by a member of the committee every three months and discussed at a meeting of the Injury Prevention Committee. Over the years, the plan changed as features of the community changed but having an implementation plan and a progress monitoring plan ensured the intervention kept on track.

Once they had obtained the first six months of results, Dula and the committee held a Community Information Forum to tell the whole community about the progress being made in changing behaviour, modifying environments, and enforcing protective legislation. Dula encouraged the community to celebrate areas of success and to make changes to the plan in areas found not to be effective in achieving the intended outcomes.

How will your group monitor the strategies they have decided to implement? It is important to plan how work is going to be monitored before the intervention is started. Talk through the various options to decide how the information that your group will need can be gathered.

Start by asking: How will you measure what is being done? How will you know what has changed? What has been the effect on fall injuries? How will the answers to these questions be recorded? Who by? How will the answers be used to improve the strategies? How long will answers need to be collected after their intervention has been finished? Where will the information be kept to help improve community interventions in the future?

Dula obtained the ethics approval and permission from relevant authorities before the group started collecting information from their community. Check with your community leader and local authority about the permissions you will need. Remember that the community is the owner of all information gathered about its members.

MODULE 3
DROWNING

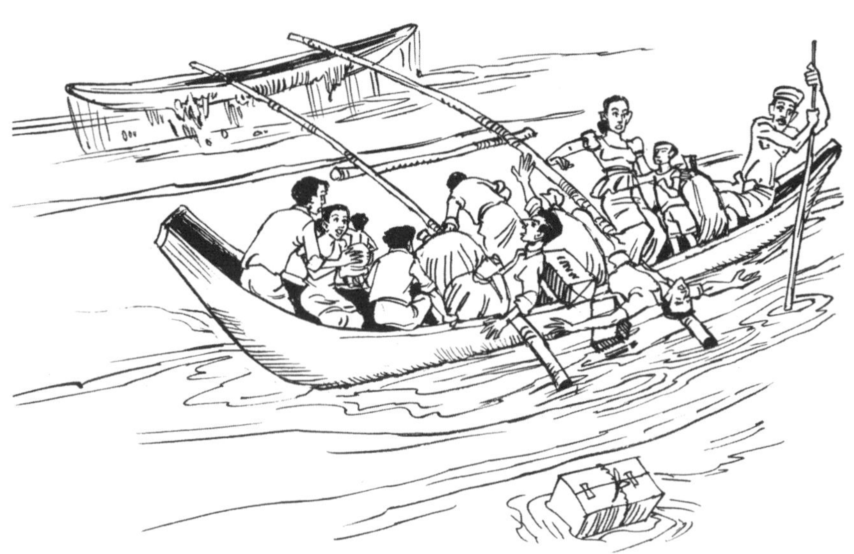

Drowning occurs when water enters the lungs and prevents the body getting the oxygen it needs to live. There are many places where people can fall into water and drown. People of all ages can drown, although young children are especially at risk. Fortunately the risk factors for drowning are well known and the ways to prevent drowning have been well tested in many communities throughout the world. By following the exercises in this chapter you can learn how to identify the risk factors for drowning. You can also learn how to develop and implement effective interventions.

Keywords: boating accidents, drowning, inhaling water, injury prevention, rivers, wells

Grasping the problem

Saman, his wife Kanthi, and one-year-old son Kumara drowned when the canoe they were in overturned in the middle of the river. Ten people had clambered on board the narrow canoe designed to carry only three.

While attending the funeral of Saman and his family, Dula felt saddened by the fact that this loss of life was unnecessary. The drownings could have been prevented. The lives could have been saved.

Dula raised her concerns about the lack of water safety in the community when she next met with the Injury Prevention Committee of Dingly. She talked about the size of the problem and about measures that had been shown to prevent drowning in other communities. The committee members recognized the need for a collaborative approach based on community knowledge and good local information. The committee decided to form a working group to find out more about the problem of drowning in Dingly and to help them work with the community to solve the problem.

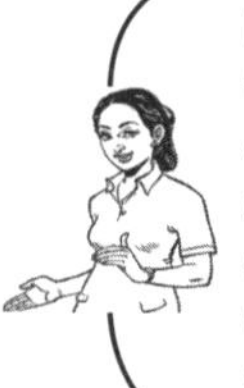

Do the members of your committee recognize the need to engage the community in solving the problem? Who are the people in your community that you believe have a role to play in the planning and implementation of interventions to prevent drowning in your community? Invite the people on your list to the next meeting of the Injury Prevention Committee to participate in a water safety working group.

http://dx.doi.org/10.3362/9781780448022.005

What is drowning?

Drowning is inhaling water, instead of oxygen, into the lungs. When water blocks the flow of air to the lungs, blood oxygen levels fall. This results in difficulty in breathing and perhaps death. The lack of oxygen can damage other important organs such as the brain, heart, and nervous system.

Where can drowning take place?

Dula asked the group to name the places where drowning can occur by identifying all the places where it was possible for someone to be underwater (or some other liquid) and breathe water or other fluid instead of air. The group's list included:

- dams;
- lakes;
- rivers and creeks;
- rice fields;
- swimming pools;
- ocean.

After some more discussion, the group realized that drowning can also occur (especially among babies and infants) in smaller bodies of water, including:

- buckets;
- baths;
- rice fields;
- drains;
- canals.

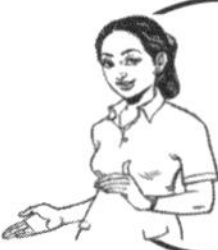

Discuss with your group the places where drowning can occur. The information from Dula's group could provide a base for your brainstorming session.

The nature and extent of the problem

Each community is different and so are its problems. Local information is needed to support decisions about prioritizing, designing and implementing interventions at the community level that will contribute to strengthening protective environments. The group realized they needed answers to the following main questions:

- Who is drowning?
- Where are the drownings happening?
- When are the drownings occurring?
- How serious are the injuries resulting from near drownings?
- How many drownings happened in the past year?
- What was happening when the person was drowned?
- Are the numbers of drownings changing over time?
- Which injuries are most significant in terms of direct costs, and social and personal harms?

By answering these questions Dula's group could decide whether drowning was a big problem in Dingly, when and where the injuries were occurring, and which groups of people were more vulnerable.

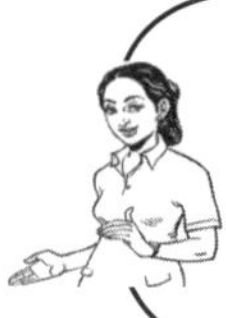

Go through the same process with your group to help them identify the questions they feel they need answered before they can move forward. Support them to use the local data and information gathered through small discussion groups with parents, fishermen and community leaders.

Dula's group drew up a list of the places and people who could be approached to provide information. The local medical clinic staff in the working group suggested the clinic would have some information. Someone suggested the police might have further information.

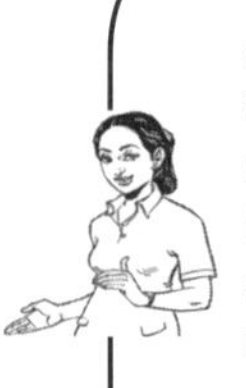

The information-gathering stage can be time consuming, but it is a very important step. Follow Dula's example to work out a way to collect the information you need. At the end of the information collection process, encourage your group to hold a public meeting in the community so they can share the information they have obtained. This will help develop support for the actions you will undertake in the future.

If you are collecting information in your community, get permission from the relevant authorities before you start.

Risk factor identification

Risk factors for drowning are the individual-, neighbourhood-, and population-level factors that increase the chance that someone goes underwater and cannot surface before they inhale water into their lungs.

Decreasing the number of drowning risk factors in Dingly could decrease the likelihood of people drowning. First, the group had to find the risk factors. Here is what they did.

Individual- and family-level risk factors for drowning

The group divided into three smaller teams, and each wrote a list of individual and family characteristics that make it more likely that someone might drown. The combined list of risk factors looked like this:

- There is lot of water around people's homes.
- It is easy for people of all ages to fall into the water.
- In some areas of water (such as wells), it is impossible to climb out.
- Many people are too young or frail to climb out of even small amounts of water.
- Many people are unable to swim to the shore if they fall into deep water.
- Some people may be drunk (intoxicated by alcohol) or unable to swim.
- Children are inquisitive and 'get into things'.
- Carers busy with many daily tasks cannot closely watch children the whole time.

The group asked Dula if the books she had been reading had identified any other things about drowning risk factors. They added Dula's suggestions to the list. The group then organized themselves into teams and arranged a series of focus groups to see if these risk factors were problems in Dingly. A focus group of mothers came up with more information about things the working group had not thought of. The team running the workshop brought these ideas back to the working group:

- Watercraft may not have adequate safety equipment and life vests.
- People often overcrowd their boats.
- The environment in or near areas where water is collected may be unsafe (slippery, uneven or unstable).
- Many people fish in unsafe conditions (such as during floods).
- Few people know about water safety measures and resuscitation of people who have inhaled the water.

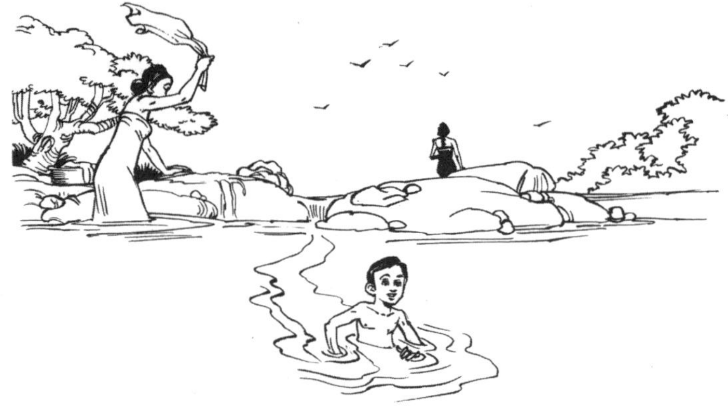

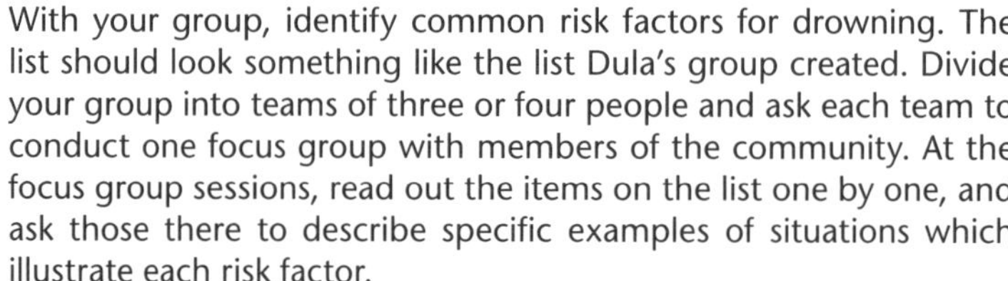

With your group, identify common risk factors for drowning. The list should look something like the list Dula's group created. Divide your group into teams of three or four people and ask each team to conduct one focus group with members of the community. At the focus group sessions, read out the items on the list one by one, and ask those there to describe specific examples of situations which illustrate each risk factor.

When all the focus group sessions have been completed, bring your group back together and put all the examples together. This information will give a good picture of the specific risk factors responsible for drowning in your community.

Neighbourhood-level risk factors for drowning

Dula next focused on helping the group identify the neighbourhood factors. She drew a map of the area on a large sheet of paper, prepared by pasting together smaller pieces of paper. This not only saved money, but also increased the active participation of all group members. Each person marked on the map all the bodies of water around Dingly where people could drown. First they included:

- natural bodies of water in the area – rivers, creeks, sea;
- other water bodies – dams , lakes, ditches.

Then they shaded in:

- areas that are frequently affected by floods.

Finally, they marked on the map:

- construction sites with water collections (e.g. barrels, tanks).

To make sure the map was accurate, Dula gave a small section of it to each of the teams of three or four that had undertaken the focus groups. Each team went to their area of Dingly to check that the map was correct and added any additional features that had not been included.

The teams put their maps back together into one large map. The working group was now confident that the map accurately represented all of the environmental risk factors for drowning in Dingly.

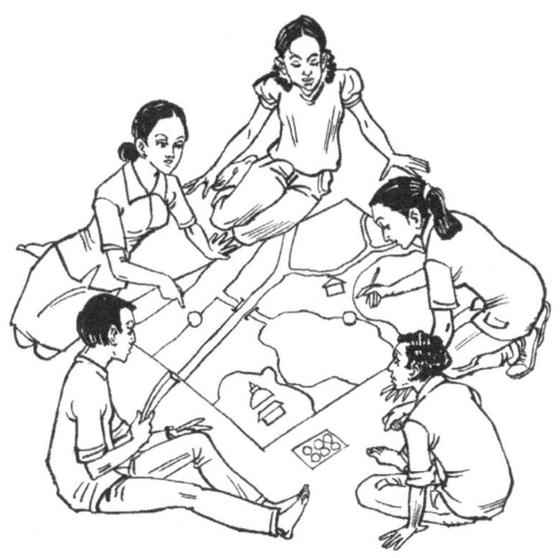

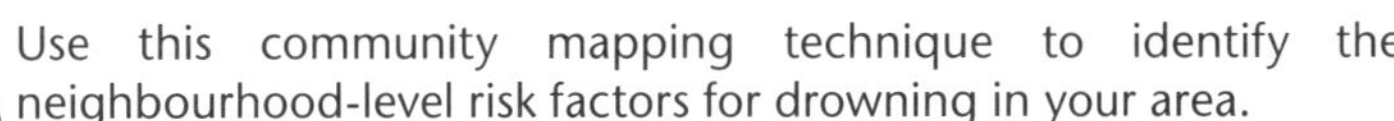
Use this community mapping technique to identify the neighbourhood-level risk factors for drowning in your area.

Population-level (structural) risk factors for drowning

Standards and regulations to promote safe daily activities associated with water-related activities are an important part of managing the risk factors for drowning. A lack of these standards and regulations is in itself a risk factor for drowning.

Dula divided the group into three teams and allocated each one of the following water-related activities.

- There are no rules and guidelines relating to maintaining standards of boats, such as the number of passengers allowed or access to life jackets.
- There are no warnings or nets to prevent swimming and washing in dangerous areas of the river.
- There are no regulations requiring village wells to be adequately covered or fenced to prevent children from falling in.

She asked each team to talk to different authorities and identify standards, policies, regulations, and laws that related to individual and neighbourhood risk factors. The group paid particular attention to community life relating to fishing in and travelling over water, and washing, bathing and swimming at home and in creeks, rivers, and oceans.

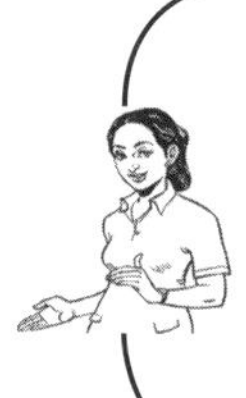

The group discussed what the teams had found. Dula challenged them to list the areas where insufficient regulation could be a population-level risk factor for drowning around Dingly. Follow the approach Dula took to identify the laws and regulations in your community that relate to safety around water. Once you have done this, ask your group to suggest laws and regulations they think need to be put in place.

The group looked at other population-level factors that were not to do with regulations and laws, but which increased the risk of drowning. They identified the following issues:

- no bridge over the river, and it was beyond the financial capacity of the community to build one;
- no warning system for natural disasters, such as floods and tsunamis;
- no danger or emergency signals;

- no lifeguards at the local swimming areas;
- lack of knowledge about immediate first aid after drowning.

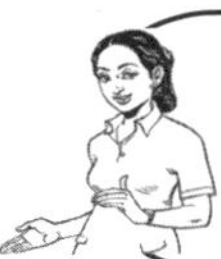

Intervention development and implementation

Setting aims for interventions

Dula's group had learnt much over the previous weeks about how to prevent drowning. They had used their existing knowledge and experience and expanded this knowledge by working together. They had been able to obtain information about the environment from direct observation, from talking to local people, and reading reports by drowning prevention experts. Dula found information through her reading and told the group about activities that had been found to be effective in promoting water safety and preventing drowning in other villages.

Now it was time for the group to work out what they wanted to achieve in Dingly. They focused their initial thinking on what they wanted to see different after the intervention. After a long discussion, one group member summarized their discussion by writing on the chart: *'Our main aim: to eliminate drowning-related deaths in Dingly within three years'*.

The group checked to see if the aim was sustainable, measurable, achievable, realistic, and time-specified (SMART).

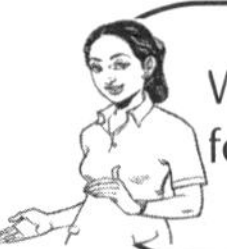

Dula's group decided to write an implementation action plan that involved the whole community in using the three strategies they knew were critical to preventing injuries and promoting safety: behaviour change, environmental modification, and enforcement of rules.

THE DINGLY DROWNING PREVENTION ACTION PLAN	
Our aim	To eliminate drowning-related deaths in Dingly within three years
Strategy 1	Increase participation in drowning prevention by people who are responsible for potential causes of drowning in Dingly
Activities	• Work with mothers, fathers and grandparents to increase supervision of children near bodies of water such as pools, rivers, and lakes • Support families to reduce the number of unprotected bodies of water around the house, either by eliminating them or by erecting childproof fences around the water • Encourage all members of the family to learn to swim • Educate people about the dangers of drinking alcohol on boats, by the river, or near other places where people could drown • Work with adult family members to encourage their safe use of watercraft and to teach their children how to behave safely around water • Encourage responsible practices in workplaces in relation to loading and use of watercraft • Support families, workplaces and schools to implement resuscitation training for all members of the community
Strategy 2	Increase the number of collaborative projects across the community designed to reduce risk factors for drowning in Dingly
Activities	• Work with property owners, builders and local government to cover or fence off all waterways from the household living space and (where possible) publicly accessible land • Where waterways cannot be fenced, clearly signpost the dangers and reduce the risk of slipping or tripping from the bank into the water • Work with manufacturers to increase the safety of the boats used in Dingly
Strategy 3	Advocate to government and international aid groups to support improvements in water-related infrastructure, and to create and enforce water safety regulations across the community
Activities	• Develop the case for funding construction of a bridge across the river • Develop the case for piping water to Dingly and closing the open water channels • Create opportunities for the community to get involved in supporting structural and legislative changes needed to ensure there are no unprotected (unfenced) water areas children can fall into • Encourage governments, community leaders, and religious leaders to set safety standards around water environments and commercial boating activity • Obtain community support for the authorities to enforce the laws and regulations that are in place

Dula reminded her group that if they could develop a plan of inter-related activities that removed the risk factors, they would be able to prevent drowning. After some discussion, the group drafted the drowning prevention action plan for discussion with the whole village (see facing page).

Putting the plan into practice

Implementing a plan is a challenge that requires the involvement and coordination of people from across the entire community. It needs support from families, but also from businesses and workplaces, and from the government and community leaders.

The group began by encouraging discussion within the community to raise awareness of the importance of the problem of drowning and the need for action. This allowed the community to be part of the solution. The group put articles in the local newspapers and spoke on local radio about the size of the problem and how much the problem could be reduced with the recommended changes. They put information on community noticeboards, and erected signs in dangerous areas warning the public of the risk of drowning. The group held public meetings in the village, and gave presentations at the schools and workplaces.

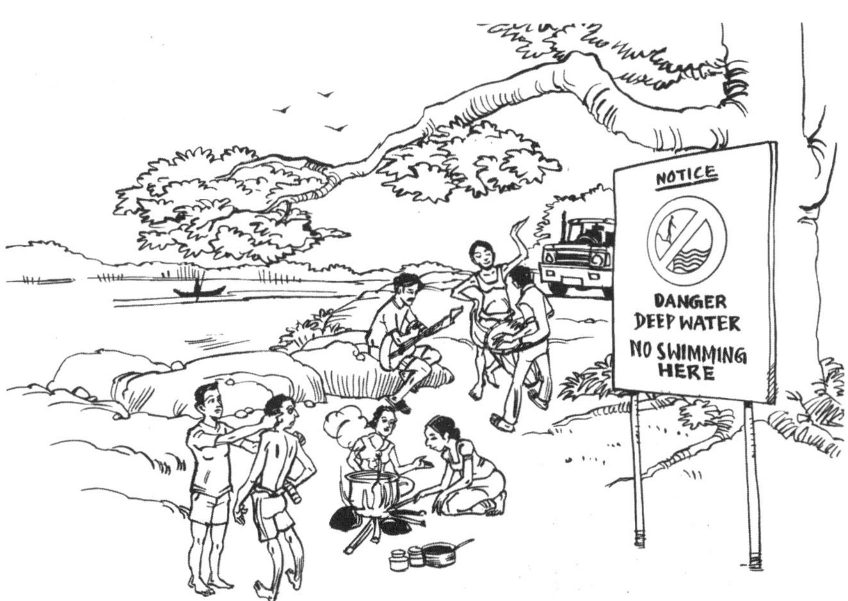

The group increased the community's willingness to become involved by providing a free service to members of the community who wanted to learn how to be safe from drowning. They developed an information and home-visiting service for parents who wanted to make their homes safe for their children. The group developed a 'learn to swim' programme that was delivered by volunteers in schools and workplaces. They worked with local suppliers to develop a cheap, effective barrier system that could be used around wells and ponds in the village. The group was able to show that if people have the right information, behaviour, and equipment, it is possible to be safer, with less chance of drowning.

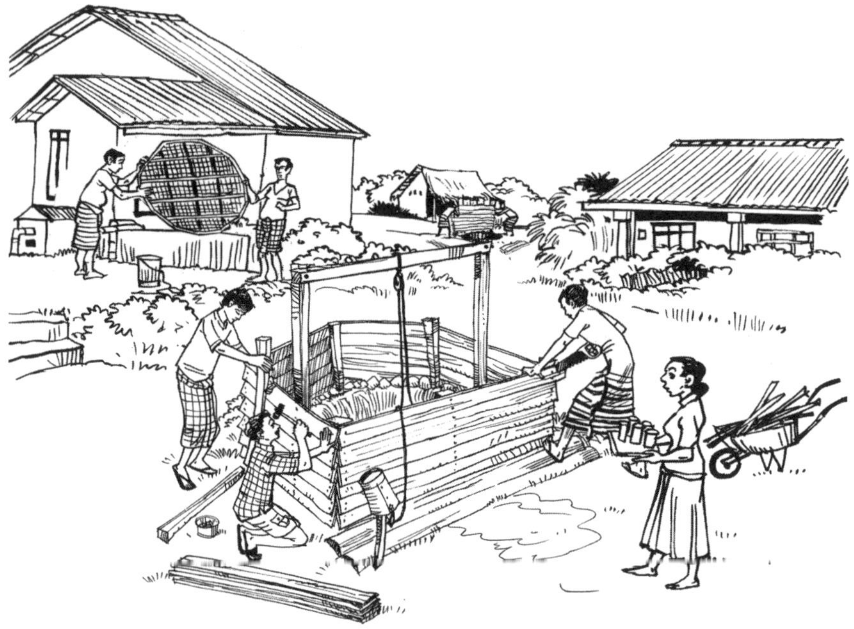

Once the community was willing to become involved in solving the drowning problem in Dingly, Dula's group was able to work through the activities listed under Strategies 1, 2 and 3 of their drowning prevention action plan.

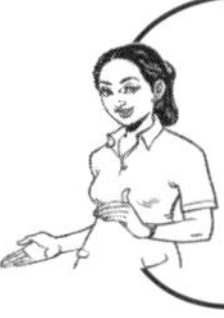

How will you engage your community in implementing your drowning prevention action plan? How are you going to change the behaviour, environment, and policies that affect your village to prevent drowning deaths?

Progress monitoring

Dula wanted to evaluate whether they had made progress towards their three-year objective during the first six months. Dula and the group developed an intervention monitoring worksheet. The worksheet was four pages long. On the first page, they recorded information that would tell them whether the activities were implemented according to their plan. On the second page, they noted whether the desired changes in the community had been achieved. On the third page, they recorded information about whether the number and severity of injuries were decreasing. On the fourth page, they collected data for the first six months of the intervention and used the results to make adjustments to their implementation plan that would improve its effectiveness. Dula's group repeated the evaluation at the end of the three years to measure the changes that were now in place.

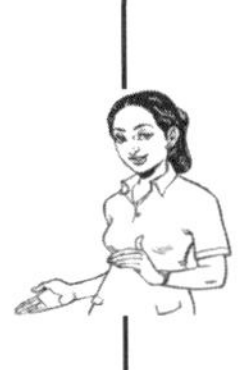

How will your group monitor the interventions that you have implemented in your area? It is important to plan the monitoring process before you start your intervention. Talk through the options with your group and ask them to think about the following questions. What activities will you undertake to prevent drowning? What are the ways you are going to measure 'what is being done', 'what has changed', and 'what effect this has had on the number of drownings'? How are these measures being defined and recorded? Is any information about these measures available from other sources that you could use in your evaluation?

MODULE 4
TRANSPORT INJURIES

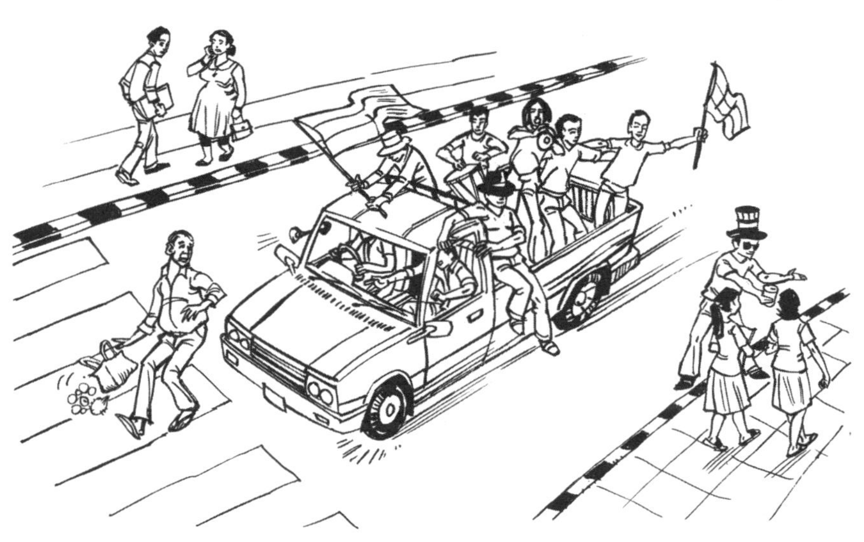

Transport injuries are a significant problem for all communities. This type of injury usually involves large amounts of kinetic energy and commonly causes serious injury and death. Ninety per cent of the world's transport injuries occur in low and middle-income countries, and this is expected to rise over the next 10 years as the number of motor vehicles on roads increases. Risk factors for transport injury relate to the transport vehicle involved, the people using the transport, and the environment in which the transport is used. The interventions also relate to these three parts of the transport system. As with all injury prevention activities, transport injury interventions involve a combination of behavioural change, environmental modification and enforcement. There is clear evidence from many communities that transport injury prevention works. This chapter helps you develop interventions that work in your community.

Keywords: injury prevention, motor vehicles, road safety, road users, roads, transport injury

Grasping the problem

Last month, the brother of one of the members of the Dingly Injury Prevention Committee was hit by a truck when he was walking by the side of the road. His right leg was so badly damaged that it had to be cut off below the knee. He has not been able to work and his family has had no income since the incident. There were seven teenagers in the truck, which was driven by a 17-year-old boy. They were coming from a school cricket match.

Two years ago, there was a train crash at the railway crossing. As usual, all the coaches of the train were crowded and hundreds of passengers were clinging to the roof and side boards. The train slammed into a crowded bus that was crossing the railway track. More than 50 people died in that crash and 150 were severely injured. Two years later, there is still no warning signal or gate at the site of the crash.

Another committee member told of a car crash in which three family members (including two children) died. The driver of the car was travelling too fast, lost control and ploughed into a crowd waiting at the side of the road for the next bus.

There were so many transport injuries that people in Dingly had started to accept death and disability caused by road and train

http://dx.doi.org/10.3362/9781780448022.006

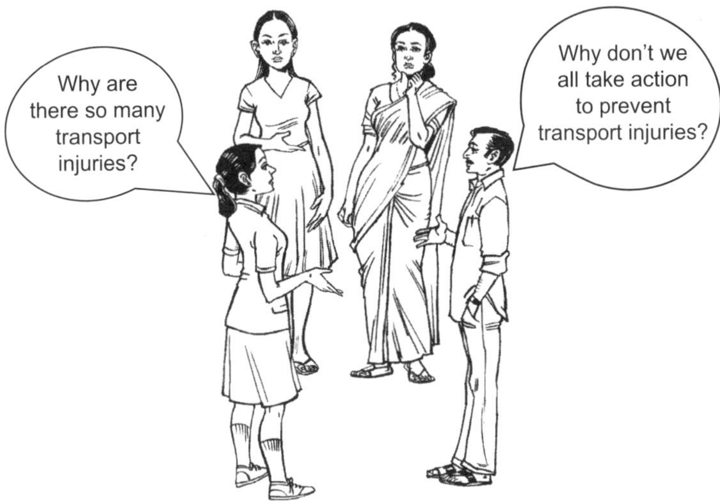

crashes as a normal part of life. However, other communities very similar to Dingly had been able to reduce the number of people being injured by changing the way people drove; the way the cars, roads, and rail crossings were made; and the way the transport environment was organized.

The committee decided to form a working group to find out more about the problem of transport injury in Dingly. The aim was to work with the community to find ways to change people's behaviour, to modify the environment, and to enforce the road safety laws and vehicle design regulations.

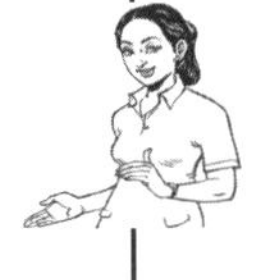

The three important messages are that: 1) transport injuries are a big problem; 2) transport injuries are preventable; and 3) there is information available from other communities about ways to prevent transport injury in your community.

Help the members of your committee understand the need to involve the community in solving the problem. Support them in seeing that changes last only if the change is made easy and people can see how it will be good for them. Who are the people in your community who could collaborate with your group to develop and implement long-lasting change? Invite all the people you think might have a role in reducing transport injuries to your next Injury Prevention Committee meeting. Invite people to share their knowledge and experience to make a difference to the people being injured on the roads and rail tracks of their community by participating in the transport injury prevention working group.

What is a transport injury?

Dula asked the group to explain what they mean by 'transport injuries' and she wrote the key words they mentioned on the blackboard. Then she put together those key words to build up the description of transport injuries.

TRANSPORT INJURY

A transport injury is the transfer of energy from a moving vehicle to a person during a collision on a public road, railway track, or footway.

What causes transport injury?

Dula asked members in her group to list the causes of transport injury. She wrote their responses on flipchart paper.

It was agreed that transport injury can be caused by the transfer of energy, such as:

- energy from a moving vehicle transferred to a pedestrian when the vehicle hits the person walking on the road or rail tracks;
- energy transferred to the drivers or passengers of the vehicles when two vehicles crash;
- energy transferred to the driver or passenger of a single vehicle when it runs off the road, hitting a roadside structure or rolling over.

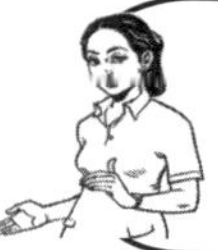

Who gets transport injuries?

Dula asked group members to think about who is involved in transport injuries. Dula asked the group members to show each other respect by raising their hand and waiting for the 'talking stick' (or other object) to be passed to him or her before they made a suggestion. She explained that no one should speak unless they

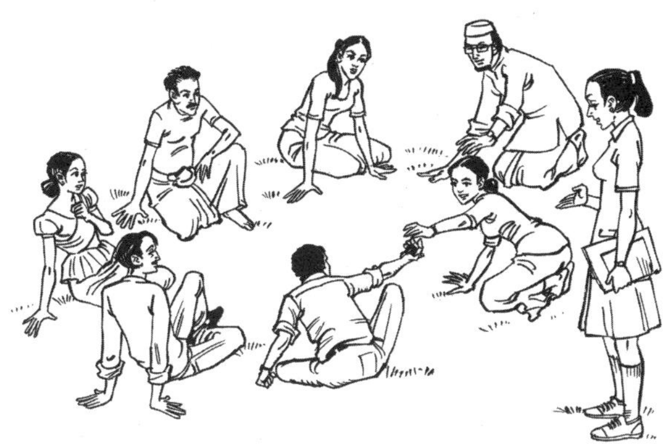

are holding the stick. The group felt this was a good idea because it gave everyone a chance to say something and also a chance to listen to others, as well as time to think about what was being said.

While they were speaking, one group member wrote down the ideas people raised. The responses included:

- people walking (pedestrians);
- people riding bikes (cyclists);
- people on motor bikes (motorcyclists);
- drivers;
- passengers of cars, rickshaws, tut tuts (vehicles);
- passengers of buses;
- passengers of trains.

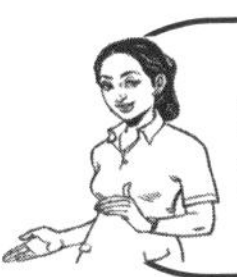

What are the outcomes of transport injuries?

Because a moving vehicle has so much energy, it can do a lot of damage to a person when this energy is released at the time of a crash.

Dula's group talked about how transport injuries affect not only the person who is injured, but also their family and their community. They wrote these potential outcomes on a flipchart.

Injured person

- head injury;
- cuts;
- disfigurement and loss of body movements;
- ongoing pain;
- damage to the skin;
- injury to other organs like liver, heart, lungs;
- broken bones;
- mental health problems;
- loss of school or working days;
- unemployment;
- death.

Family members

- cost for treatment;
- problems caring for the injured;
- loss of family income;
- loss of the care and support given by the injured person;
- emotional trauma.

Community

- cost for emergency care;
- cost for prolonged hospitalizations;
- cost for rehabilitation;
- cost of property damage.

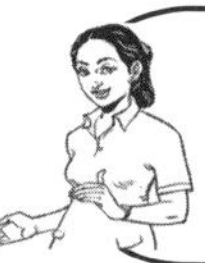

Conduct a brainstorming session with your group to suggest outcomes of transport crashes and ask one group member to write them on the blackboard or flipchart.

The nature and extent of the problem

Dula asked her group to find out more about the transport injury problem in Dingly. She asked them to find out where most injuries happened, what time of day most injuries happened, and which people (age, male or female, district) were most at risk.

The group found this difficult because they did not have exact information. They only had stories. They decided that it would be a good idea to do a survey of the transport situation so they could get accurate details.

To get a clear picture of the transport injury problem in Dingly, the group decided they needed answers to the following questions: Who is being injured? Where are the injuries occurring? When are the injuries occurring? How serious are the injuries? How many injuries have happened? Under what circumstances are injuries occurring? Are rates of injury changing over time? Which injuries do the most harm in terms of direct costs, and social and personal outcomes?

Dula helped the group identify the steps they had to follow to do their survey, as well as some things to think about before they got started.

Here are some key points to think about when planning a field survey to describe the extent and the risk factors for transport injuries in your area.

- Where will you conduct the survey? This may be the local health area, local police area, or local government district.
- How will you collect the data? Should you gather information on transport injuries by asking people questions, or should you get the data from existing records? Is it practical to ask people to fill out forms themselves?
- How long will the data be collected? Should it be for just a short period, such as a few weeks, or should you set up a system that goes on collecting data or only at regular intervals?
- What places do you need to visit to collect data? Is the survey to be completed by staff and patients at the hospital, or people at the police station, insurance companies, or in their homes? Is information from newspapers and newsletters useful?
- What permission is needed to collect the data? As you are collecting information about your community, you need to get permission from the relevant authorities. You also need to get permission from the people you are questioning.
- How do you get the money needed to do a survey? Who can you approach to get funding?
- How will the data be understood? You need to find someone who can tell you what the data means; that is, what information

it gives you to help your group know where, when and how changes are most urgently needed. You might be able to get help with this from government departments, aid agencies, or perhaps the maths teacher at the local high school.

- How will the data be presented? You will need to make the data as easy as possible for people to understand. Data is often best presented using graphs and diagrams.
- How will the findings be shared with others? The information you have will be most useful if it reaches as many people as possible. Perhaps you can hold community presentations to share the information you have gathered, and arrange meetings with community leaders and government authorities to present the findings of your survey.

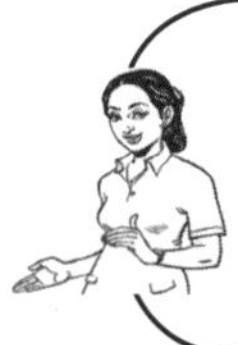

Go through the same process with your group to work out the size of the problem in your community, which groups of people are more at risk, and when and where the injuries are occurring. Check with your local community leaders and authorities about getting permission to collect the data.

Risk factor identification

Individual- and family-level risk factors for transport injuries

When we are talking about transport injury, individual-level risk factors relate to the people involved: for example, pedestrians, cyclists, motorcyclists, drivers, occupants of vehicles, buses, or trains (passengers). People in each of these groups have different risks of being injured in a crash.

One person from the group put up her hand to ask, 'Dula, these people are grouped together by the way they use the road or public transport. But children are in all the groups (except motorcyclists and drivers). I think they are an "at risk" group too.'

Other members of the group then started to suggest other groupings of people who might have an increased risk of being in a transport crash.

'I think older people who try to drive might be more at risk of injury,' said one. Another said, 'Yes, but most of the transport injuries I know about are from car crashes caused by young male drivers. Is being young a risk factor for transport injury?'

Dula's group added three more risk categories to their flipchart:

* children;
* young males;
* older drivers.

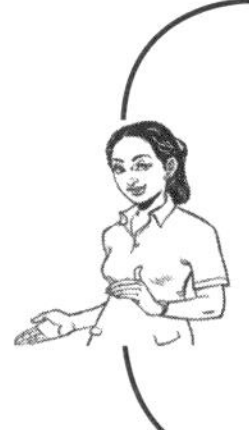

In Dula's group, this exercise created a lot of discussion and the conversation lasted a long time. People were interested in all the different types of transport users who were at risk of injury. Encourage a similar discussion with your group to identify people at risk of transport injuries. Pass around a 'talking stick', a stone or some other object so everyone has a say. Ask one group member to write the responses on the flipchart so that everyone can see and think about them.

Dula asked her group to think about other risk factors for transport injury. She suggested that the group take each road user group, one by one, and list all the risk factors that relate to that group of road users. She observed that most individual factors that increased people's risk of transport injury related to the transport users' behaviour.

She divided her group into smaller teams of three or four and asked members of the small teams to discuss the issues. When they came back into one group, they combined their lists for each type of transport user, and the main types of user behaviour that increase people's risk of having a transport-related injury. This is what their combined list looked like:

Pedestrians

* alcohol;
* using the road or train tracks as a footpath;
* not crossing the road at designated pedestrian crossings;
* trying to get across the road or rail crossing before a car or train.

Drivers

* speeding;
* driving when under the influence of alcohol;

- driving when too tired;
- being distracted while driving (e.g. by mobile phones or children);
- not wearing a seatbelt;
- trying to beat the oncoming train to the rail crossing;
- not obeying the road rules.

Cyclists

- not wearing a helmet;
- not wearing bright, reflective clothing;
- speeding;
- riding when under the influence of alcohol;
- riding when too tired;
- being distracted while riding (e.g. by mobile phones or children);
- not obeying the road rules.

Passengers in cars and buses and trains

- not wearing seatbelts;
- overcrowding;
- hanging on the outside of the vehicles.

Children

- playing on the road or train tracks;
- not looking when crossing the road or train tracks;
- not being big enough to be seen or to get themselves out of danger;
- not being properly restrained in vehicles.

Young males

- being overconfident in their driving abilities;
- driving too fast;
- leaving too little room for error;
- being distracted by music, passengers, or a mobile phone.

Older drivers

- not being able to see or react quickly to other vehicles;
- not being aware of the traffic when crossing the road;
- being too frail to survive if involved in a crash.

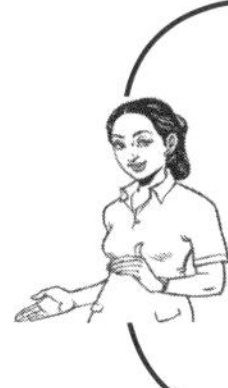

Divide your group into small teams to discuss the types of behaviour that increase people's risk of injury. It is important for you to make sure someone from each small team writes down the main points, so that when you get your whole group together you will be able to create a summary list. You will be able to use this when talking to others about the problem of transport injury.

Neighbourhood-level risk factors for transport injuries

Dula then asked a question that really surprised her group: 'How many of you have never made even the smallest mistake when you have tried to do something complicated?' No one put their hand up; everyone had fumbled or slipped or bumped into something when going about their daily activities.

Dula pointed out that people driving cars or walking or riding buses and trains make mistakes too. But, because so much energy is carried in a moving vehicle, these little mistakes can result in serious injuries and death.

Many people think that all transport injuries can be prevented by telling people to drive more carefully. A much better result can be achieved if you address the neighbourhood risk factors linked to roads/rail tracks and vehicles. Then, if road users make little mistakes, they should not be seriously injured.

Dula and her group decided to walk around the village and list all the places where the roads and train tracks were not safe. They started by drawing a map of Dingly on a large piece of paper. They divided the paper into four pieces and the group into four teams, and gave one piece of the map to each team. Each team went to the part of Dingly represented on their piece of the map and listed the risk factors related to roads and train tracks.

They looked at the surface of the road and noted the big holes and broken edges that would make cars crash. They looked at how wide the road was for the number of vehicles that travelled on it. They noted whether vehicles going in both directions could safely pass each other. They looked at how steep the road was. They looked for line markings on the road to show where the cars should drive. They looked for sharp corners, for barriers that prevented vehicles going off the road, and for protection in the middle of the road that stopped cars crossing the road into oncoming traffic. They checked how the people crossed the road and whether there were paths for people to walk beside the road. They checked whether drivers could see people walking or other cars, or whether there were things that blocked their view. Were there any street lights? They looked at speed limit signs in the village. The team members marked everything they saw on their part of the map.

When the teams came back, they put together the four pieces of the Dingly map and then divided into teams again to discuss the many problems they had found with the Dingly road system.

There were tractors on the road, mixed with push bikes and goats, and motor bikes and cars. None of the cars and the motor bikes in Dingly had the high-quality safety features that were now found in cars used in many towns and cities in other parts of the world. There were few fitted seatbelts, no airbags, no roll protection reinforcement. Most of the vehicles in Dingly were old and in need of repair. The village did not have an ambulance service or a big hospital that was equipped to provide trauma care.

At the end of these discussions, the group came together to list the neighbourhood-level risk factors that would need to be addressed to reduce transport injury in Dingly.

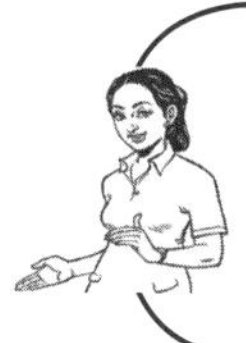

Divide your group into four teams. Use the approach Dula used to assess your community for neighbourhood-level risk factors for transport injury. At the end of the exercise bring everyone together and discuss the lists the teams have created. See if you can get more suggestions from the whole group to add to the list.

Population-level (structural) risk factors for transport injuries

Dula asked her group to tell her why cars were not safe, why the design of the roads was not good, and why people often drove too fast, too tired, and too drunk. This was where Dula's group started to get really excited. People suggested that safe cars were not available, and that the government did not build the right kind of environment so that people could get around safety. They said there should be better regulations to stop people behaving badly on the road and that the police should enforce these laws. They agreed that the people of Dingly needed to understand the importance of following proper road rules and allow the police to do their job properly.

Dula explained a lot of what they were talking about was called 'transport safety management'. Road users are simply one part of the transport system. The group talked about how many people across the full range of public and private, government and industry organizations had a part to play in designing, building and maintaining the transport system. They agreed that if these people managed the whole system well, people following the rules and using the transport system safely would not suffer serious injury.

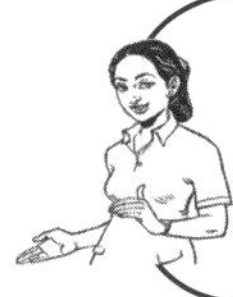

Ask your group to list the people who have a part to play in designing, building and managing the transport systems. What does your group think are the transport safety management factors that make transport users safe?

Intervention development and implementation

Setting aims for interventions

Thinking about what they had learnt, Dula and the group talked about the exact actions needed to solve the problem of transport injury in Dingly. They wanted their proposed intervention to be sustainable, measurable, achievable, realistic, and time-specified. After looking at all the information they had written on the flipchart, the group agreed that the aim of their intervention was *to reduce transport-related injuries and deaths in Dingly by 10 per cent each year for the next five years.*

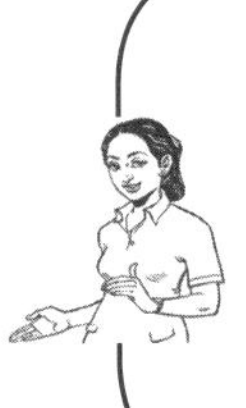

Encourage your group to be clear about what they must do to make change happen and to continue into the future. Help them create a transport injury prevention action plan that focuses on interventions that will reduce the risk factors in their community. Encourage them to collaborate, right from the start of their planning, with those who can assist them in improving the transport safety of their district. Help them to test whether their plans are doable and will support the changes they want to bring about in the everyday life of your community.

Dula's group drafted an action plan for discussion with the whole village.

THE DINGLY TRANSPORT INJURY PREVENTION ACTION PLAN	
Our aim	To reduce transport injuries and deaths in Dingly by 10 per cent each year for the next five years
Strategy 1 *Activities*	Improve road-user behaviour in Dingly • Work with others from across your community to find ways to raise awareness about safe road use in all age groups • Support parents and school teachers to teach children and young people how to safely cross roads and train tracks • Work with garage owners to run workshops for young people to learn about safe road behaviour and how to look after their car or motorbike
Strategy 2 *Activities*	Improve safety of the vehicles and transport environment in Dingly • Work with local business owners and aid agencies to establish a low-cost, safe bus service in Dingly • Encourage schools to have bright uniforms so children can be seen more easily on the way to and from school • Work with aid agencies to support families to access and use safer vehicles, motorcycle helmets, child car seats, and reflective clothing through low-interest loans • Work with local authorities to advocate road crossings, footpaths, bike lanes, and better designed intersections • Work with local shop owners to make it easier to buy affordable personal safety clothing and equipment • Work with local councils and governments to improve the roads, road crossings, bike paths, pedestrian walkways and paths • Work with local business owners and aid agencies to establish a low-cost, safe bus service in Dingly

Strategy 3
 	
Activities
	Advocate for the improvement of laws and regulations relating to transport safety, the enforcement of these laws and the overall safety management of the transport system
	• Advocate for:
	  – better management of the roads and train lines
	  – better built and maintained roads and trains lines
	  – more regular buses and trains
	  – improved driver licensing procedures
	  – increased enforcement of safe road user behaviour
	  – improved regulation around the safety of heavy vehicles and commercial transport
	  – stricter safety requirements for locally manufactured and imported vehicles

Putting the plan into practice

Dula's group talked about how they would put their transport injury prevention action plan in place. After a lot of discussion and sharing of ideas, the group agreed that they would launch the plan at a safe transport festival that would involve the whole village. They thought this would be the best way to:

- raise understanding in all villagers that everyone has a role to play in preventing transport injuries in Dingly;
- gain approval of the draft action plan and gather support across the community to see activities implemented over the next five years;
- commence implementing Strategy 1.

Dula pointed out that when planning the festival it was important the committee ensured its key messages were clear and delivered to people in a number of different and fun ways, such as presentations, games, puppets, street theatre, and demonstrations.

They agreed that the important messages of the day were designed to increase the number of people who had a better understanding of the importance of:

- obeying the road rules;
- wearing seatbelts;
- not drinking alcohol before driving;
- not driving faster than the speed limit;
- wearing bike helmets;
- not driving when tired;
- not using mobile phones while driving.

The group decided that once the Strategy 1 activities were accepted by the community, then the activities under Strategies 2 and 3 of their action plan could be more easily developed and put in place. The big advantage the group saw in this staged approach was that successes in the first stage would reinforce the community's commitment and encourage them to continue with the more challenging activities listed under Strategies 2 and 3.

The safe transport festival was a special day for Dula and the group. They organized an opening ceremony and invited the members of the local council, parliament, representatives from non-government organizations (NGOs), local charity groups, and media. A large number of villagers gathered for the opening. The council leader gave the opening speech. Dula presented the information they had gathered from their survey about how big the road safety problem was in Dingly. Other members of the group explained how the risk factors they had identified in the village may lead to more transport injuries in the future. One group member spoke about measures that should be taken by government authorities and other organizations to reduce transport injuries in Dingly, but he also stressed that there were many things that every person living in Dingly could do immediately to help keep themselves, their loved ones, and their neighbours safer on the roads. After the opening talks, the festival carried on all day.

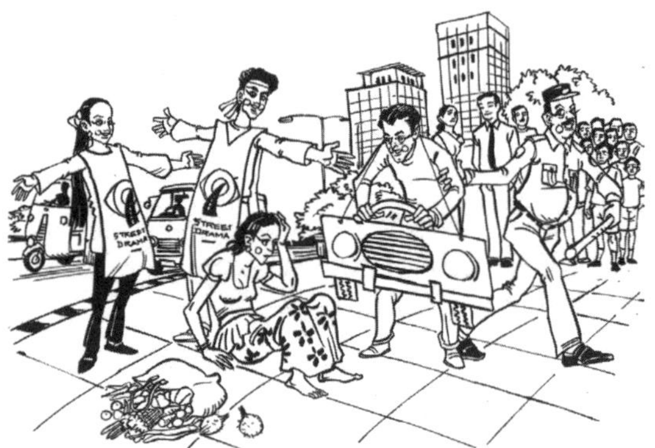

The festival included a street play on road safety performed by the youth society of the village

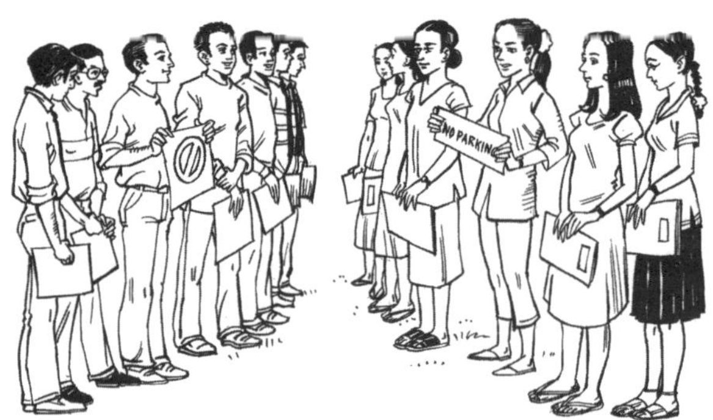

The road sign matching game was popular among people of all ages

Officers from the village police station demonstrated safe use of bicycle helmets, the rules when riding a bicycle, and how to cross the road safely. One officer gave this information to young men of the village, while another spoke to parents and another to older members of the community. One of the local primary school teachers used puppets to give the same information to young children. This was done because the committee realized that each of these groups used the roads and trains differently and needed different information to enable them to be safe transport users.

The police also provided a demonstration of the damage done to the car and the driver, and any passengers, not wearing seatbelts when a car crashes into a brick wall at moderate speed. The officers used old dummies as the driver and passengers and a car that had been taken from its owner after dangerous driving.

The committee arranged with local suppliers of helmets that meet the national safety standards to sell them at the festival at lower prices to enable more people to buy them.

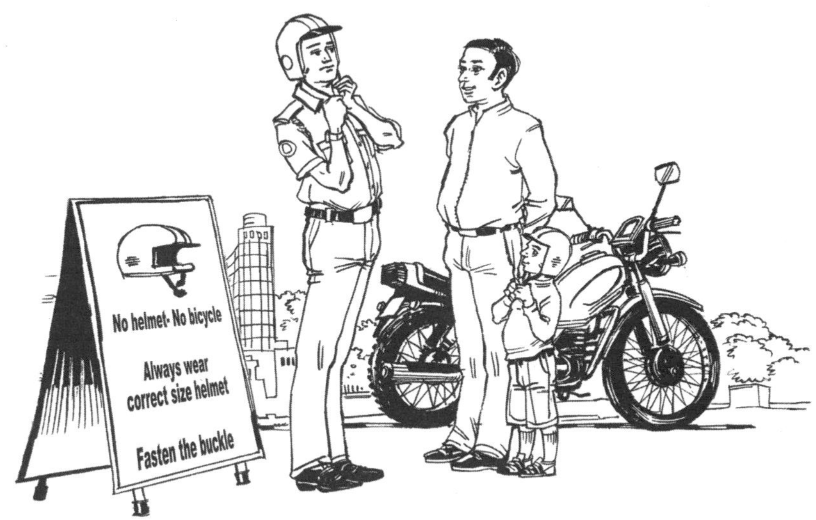

Dula invited the mobile health education unit of the health department to the festival and they showed a video on road safety. The local child health nurse talked to parents about the importance of making sure the strap on their child's motorbike helmet was done up properly.

All these activities provided people with many ways to hear the important safety promotion and injury prevention messages of the day.

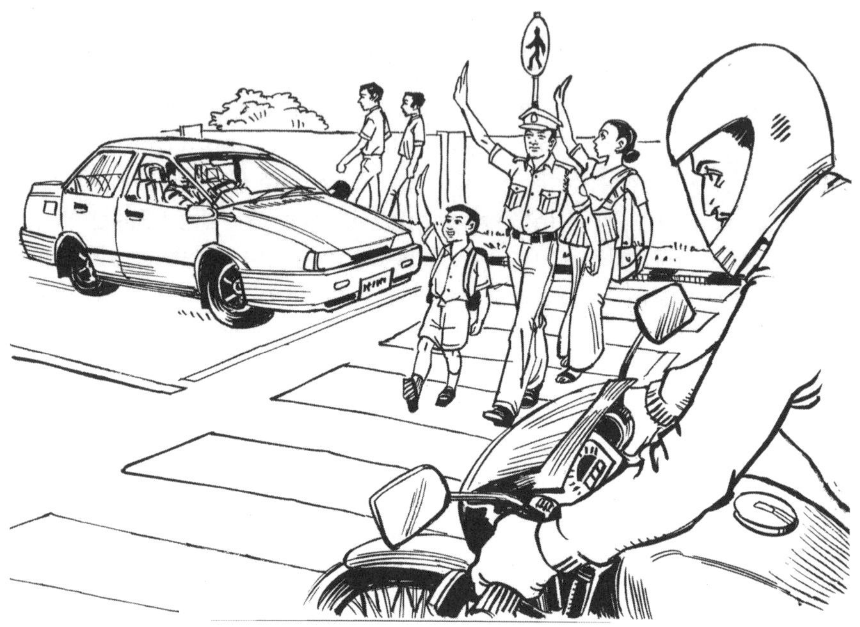

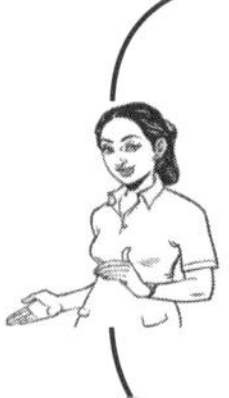

Dula sought support from other government resources such as police officers and the health education unit to make this event successful. Would it be useful to gather people together to hold a similar community event in your community? If so, encourage people in your community to decide on, plan, and carry out activities for the festival. Work with your group on other resources they could collaborate with to raise awareness of road safety.

Next steps

After the festival, the transport injury prevention working group continued to promote discussions about ways to improve road safety at community meetings and public events, and in the newspapers and on the radio. The committee worked with police to build community support for increased enforcement of road safety regulations and road rules. In particular, they focused their efforts on pedestrian behaviour, driving speed, alcohol, and the wearing of seatbelts. People were encouraged to believe they were being irresponsible if they did not obey the laws relating to road safety. People were made by their family and friends to feel ashamed if they put other people at risk of injury by their behaviour. The local primary school added a brightly coloured sash to its uniform to help make it easier to see young students walking to and from school. A culture started to grow that supported safe behaviour.

To help people obey the rules, the committee worked with manufacturers and NGOs to provide safety equipment such as low-cost bicycle helmets to people of low income.

Physical changes were also made to Dingly. These included the building of a rail gate at the railway crossing, speed humps and pedestrian crossings, repair and replacement of old or damaged road signs, and setting up of school traffic safety zones.

The committee worked with the people and organizations involved in designing, building and maintaining the transport safety system. They used the data and information they had gathered to identify the areas where safety could be improved and the people responsible for the each part of the system. The committee gave a presentation to the government department in charge of building roads, explaining the safety features that their research showed needed to be included in any new roads. They worked with the government to improve the footpaths beside the roads and increase the number of safe crossings for pedestrians. Importantly, the committee convinced the government to decrease the speed limits in built-up areas where large numbers of people lived, and near shops and schools.

The committee presented the evidence they had gathered to the people responsible for motor vehicle standards about the number of lives that could be saved by improving the quality of vehicles in Dingly.

Using these methods the Dingly road safety committee continued to lobby for, and support, improved road safety management in their village. Dula and the group planned several interventions over the years related to behavioural changes, environmental modifications and regulation and enforcement activities to reduce transport-related death and injuries in Dingly. Each intervention built on the things that worked and they changed the things that did not.

As a result of the working group's efforts, most people in Dingly became aware of the problem of transport injuries and road safety measures. They started to demand that the authorities provide them with a safer environment and most importantly they started to change the way they and their loved ones used the roads and transport system.

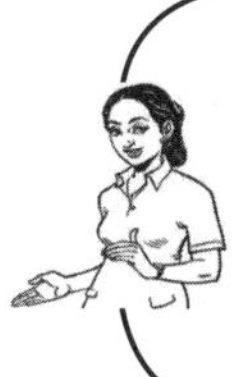

Work with your group to set aims for interventions guided by the data and information they have gathered about the transport injuries in their community and research done in other communities. What are the three strategies seen to be needed in your transport injury prevention action plan to make a difference to the number and severity of transport injuries in your community?

Progress monitoring

Dula wanted to evaluate whether they had made progress during the first six months towards their three-year aim. Dula and the group developed an intervention monitoring worksheet to give them the evidence they needed to check how useful the activities under Strategy 1 appeared to be in improving road user behaviour in Dingly.

The worksheet was four pages long. On the first page, they recorded information that would tell them whether the activities were implemented according to their plan. On the second page, they noted whether the desired changes in the community had been achieved. On the third page, they recorded information about whether the number and severity of injuries were decreasing. These questions were useful to monitor the effect of the strategies and to provide additional information that could be used to adapt the strategies as the needs of the community changed. On the fourth page, they collected data for the first six months and used the results to make adjustments to their implementation plan to improve effectiveness of the activities. Dula's group repeated the evaluation at the end of the three years of their project to measure the changes that had been achieved.

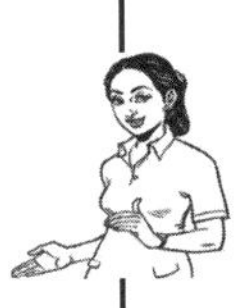

How are you going to monitor the interventions that your group has implemented in your area? Use the following prompts to encourage your group to think about what steps to take.

What does the information tell you about the interventions that need to be put in place to prevent transport injuries? What must be done now, in the next three months, and in the next twelve months? Suggest ways you will use to measure 'what is being done?', 'what has changed?', and 'what changes in transport injuries have resulted?' How are these measures being defined and recorded? Is there information available from other sources that you could use in your evaluation?

Dula obtained the ethics approval and permission from her community leaders and relevant authorities before the group started collecting information from their community. Check with your local authority to find out which permissions you need.

MODULE 5
POISONING

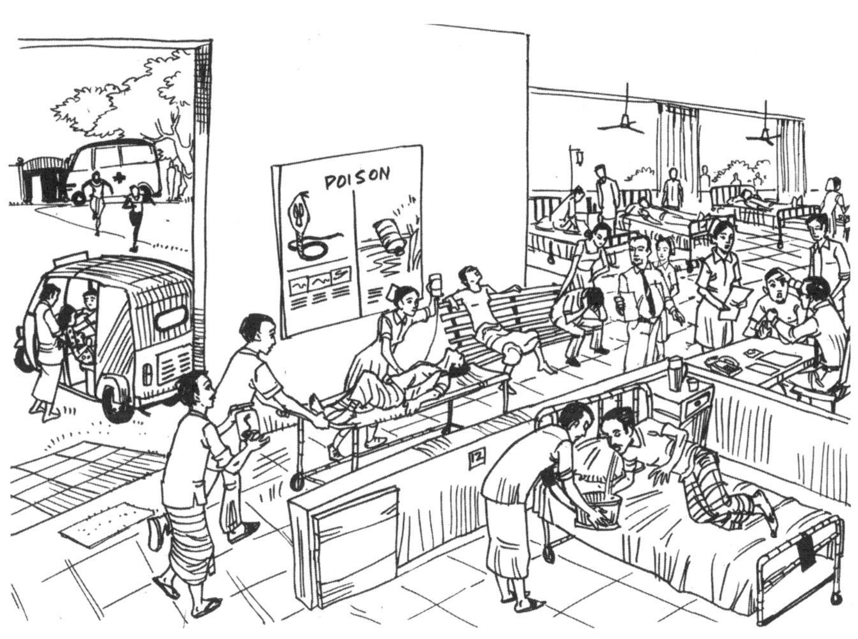

Poisoning is injury or death following exposure to chemical energy from toxic substances (poisons). Poisons can be found everywhere, including houses, sheds, workshops, and farms. Many plants around us are poisonous if eaten. It is important to learn what is and what is not poisonous. This chapter presents exercises to help you identify poisons and explore the factors in your community that increase the risk of people being poisoned. Once you have learned about the risk factors for poisoning, interventions to prevent people being exposed to poisons are simply developed and easily implemented. This chapter provides examples to help you develop action plans for reducing the problem in your community.

Keywords: chemicals, cleaning agents, ingestion, injury prevention, poisoning, sprays

Grasping the problem

It is the paddy harvesting season in Dingly village. Over recent weeks, since harvesting began, the village doctor has noticed there have been more admissions to the hospital for both pesticide poisoning and snake bites. The doctor was so concerned about the number of poisonings he approached Dula to see if she was able to help.

Dula brought the doctor's request to the attention of the Dingly Injury Prevention Committee. Each committee member talked about their experiences with poisoning and what they knew about the issues with how and why poisons were used in homes, farms, and businesses. It was clear that there were a range of different poisons and ways people could be poisoned. While members of the committee were not aware of many deaths from poisoning in their village, they did know of many people who had become sick. Most deaths they had heard about were among young children who drank things that were dangerous.

The committee decided they needed to form a working group to find out more about the problem of poisoning injury in Dingly.

http://dx.doi.org/10.3362/9781780448022.007

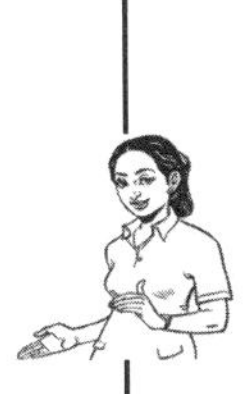

Dula, the community worker, has a good relationship with the village doctor. Because of this, the sudden increase in the number of poisonings was recognized at an early stage and people started to act. How do you communicate as the community worker with the hospital staff in your area? Who do you need to build partnerships with to enable you to respond quickly to new risks to your community?

Do the members of your committee consider poisoning to be a problem in your community? Who are the people who could help your committee develop and implement programmes? Invite all the people you think might be interested in helping to the next Injury Prevention Committee meeting, with the aim of forming a poisoning prevention working group.

What is poisoning? What can cause poisoning?

At the first meeting of the working group, Dula invited everyone to brainstorm what they understood by the word 'poisoning'. Group members went back to their basic definition of injury to help them come up with a clear definition of what they meant by 'poisoning'. This is what the group finally ended up agreeing to and wrote up on flipchart paper.

POISONING

Poisoning is injury or death following exposure to harmful or toxic substances (poisons).

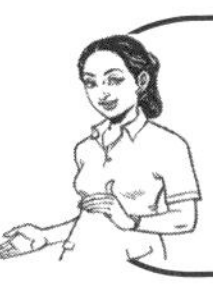

Remind your group of the basic definition of injury and ask them to come up with a definition of poisoning that looks like the one Dula's group wrote down.

What are some common poisons?

The worrying thing about poisons is that they are often used as part of daily life. They can be found everywhere: in the house, in sheds, in workshops, on farms.

Poisons generally do not cause harm if used properly, but care needs to be taken to make sure they are in fact used properly. To illustrate this, Dula put a bottle of cleaning fluid on the table and said, 'If you wash the dishes with this, it is perfectly safe. If a child drinks it, the child could die.' Then she put a bottle of paraffin on the table and said, 'Many of you use this fluid for cooking every day. If a child drinks this the child could die.' Some members of the group had not realized that cooking and cleaning fluids were poisons.

It is important to know what is a poison and what it is not. The group set out to write a list of all the common things in Dingly that are poisons. This is the list they wrote:

- chemicals used in and around house, garden, workplace, and farm, such as pesticides, animal bait, cleaning agents;
- harmful gases, smoke, fumes in the environment;
- medications and drugs;
- venoms of animals like snakes, scorpions, spiders and fish;
- essential oils;
- sap from plants.

As well as knowing what is and what is not a poison, it is important to know how these poisons can be used safely and how they could be dangerous. Different poisons can cause harm different ways. They can get into the body by:

- ingestion (eating or drinking);
- inhalation (breathing);
- absorption (contact through skin);
- injection (bite or sting of animals, needle prick, tattooing).

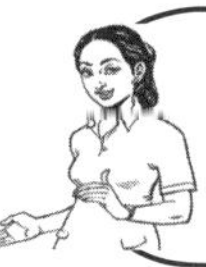

What are the outcomes of poisoning?

Different poisons can affect the body in different ways. Dula divided the group into three teams and asked each team to discuss the outcomes of poisoning for:

- the injured individual;
- family members;
- the community.

The teams came back together to share their views. One member wrote them on flipchart paper.

Injured person

- skin irritation, blisters, burns;
- pain and swelling;
- damage to the organs such as lungs, eyes, heart, kidneys and liver;
- damage to muscles and nerves;
- mental health problems;
- loss of school or working days;
- unemployment;
- death.

Family members

- cost of treatment;
- problems caring for the patient;
- loss of family income;
- no longer getting the care and support given by the injured;
- emotional trauma.

Community

- cost for emergency care;
- cost for prolonged hospitalizations;
- cost for rehabilitation.

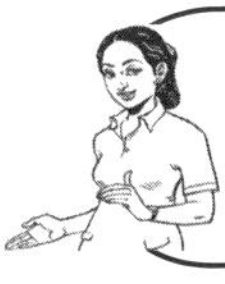

Conduct a discussion session on 'outcomes of poisoning' with your group.

The nature and extent of the problem

Dula's group had learnt what poisoning was, how it affected people, and what the broader effects can be. Now, they wanted to find out how big a problem poisoning was for Dingly.

They wanted to know:

- Who is being poisoned?
- Where are the poisonings occurring?

- When are the poisonings happening?
- How serious are the injuries caused by poisoning?
- How many poisonings have happened in the past year?
- What was happening when the person was poisoned?
- Are the numbers of poisonings changing over time?
- Which poisonings are most significant in terms of direct costs, social and personal harms?

Dula asked everyone to think about these questions and suggest how they would find the answers they needed. The main information sources suggested were the hospital or emergency department records, school records, workplace accident records. Some people felt that household surveys would be useful. The group designed a process for obtaining the information they needed using a combination of these approaches.

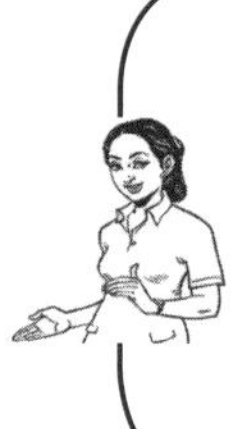

Is poisoning a big problem in your community? Does it cause lots of hospital visits or just a few? Does it cause lots of deaths or just a few? How would you know how big a problem poisoning is in your area? Go through the same process as Dula's group to measure the size of the problem in your community and work out which groups of people are more at risk of poisoning, and when and where the poisonings are happening. Did you find that most of the poisonings in your village were among young children and workers?

Risk factor identification

Individual- and family-level risk factors for poisoning

Dula and her group started talking about things that are kept in the house that can be poisonous. There are many cleaning agents that are harmful, as well as medicines, petrol, essential oils, and sprays for weeds and insects. When these are stored within reach of small children, they can be very dangerous. If medicines and potentially harmful fluids are stored in ways that disguise what they are, they can be swallowed by mistake.

Dula's group summarized the individual-/family-level risk factors they had discussed:

- poisons not out of reach of children;
- poisons not kept in a locked cupboard;

- storage of poisons with food or in food containers;
- not using child-resistant packages;
- snakes, scorpions and spiders in the house;
- bringing poisons to the home from the workplace by mistake (e.g. not changing clothes after working).

Neighbourhood-level risk factors for poisoning

Dula and the group then set off for a 'walk and talk' to identify neighbourhood-level risk factors for poisoning in Dingly village. The group divided into small teams and walked around the different parts of the village. They met the villagers and talked with them about the problem. They visited houses, factories and farms.

Following the walk, the teams gathered to share their findings. Each group presented their findings to the others, then they wrote them on the flipchart.

- The village rubbish dump had open packets and tins of poisons lying around.
- Storage sheds in the village had poisons that could be found by people just wandering by.
- Many plants in the street and village parks were poisonous.
- Footpaths in the village were covered with grass, providing hiding space to snakes.
- Pesticides, detergents, and medications were stored with food at the grocery stores.
- Workers were not wearing protective clothing when spraying pesticides and insecticides on crops in rural areas.
- Council and farm workers were not following the correct procedure when spraying insecticides and pesticides, causing the general public to be exposed to the spray.

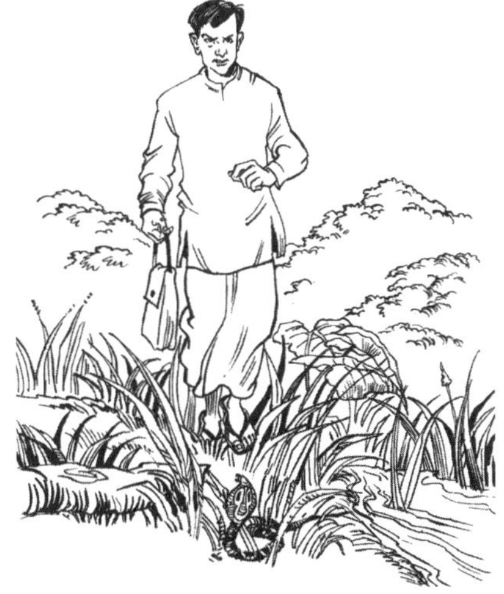

- Workers were unaware of safety precautions and the danger of poisons.
- The river where some people got their drinking water was downstream from where a factory regularly spilled poisonous waste.

Population-level risk factors for poisoning

Because most poisonings in Dingly were among young children or were a result of a problem at a factory or workplace, the group focused on looking at what was happening that led to these poisonings. They saw that there was a tolerance by authorities of bad practice in the use, storage and disposal of poisons.

There were no laws (or no enforcement of laws) relating to:

- child-resistant closures on all poison containers;
- accurate labelling of containers in which poisons and toxic substances were sold;
- readable descriptions and instructions on the poison bottles (e.g. they were sometimes written in small letters or another language);
- safe workplace practices in relation to storage and use of poisonous substances.

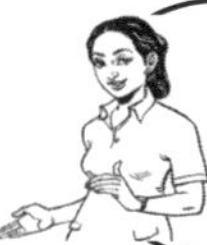

Plan a field visit with your group to identify the risk factors for poisoning in your community. Group the risk factors into individual, neighbourhood and population levels.

Intervention development and implementation

Setting aims for interventions

Once the working group had all the data and information they needed, they quickly settled on the aim of their poisoning prevention intervention. They decided they wanted: *to reduce hospitalizations and deaths from poisoning in Dingly by 10 per cent each year for the next five years.*

Dula's group drafted the following action plan for discussion with the whole village.

THE DINGLY POISONING PREVENTION ACTION PLAN	
Our aim	To reduce hospitalizations and deaths from poisoning in Dingly by 10 per cent each year for the next five years
Strategy 1	Increase participation in preventive activities by people involved with the causes of major poisoning-related injuries and deaths in Dingly
Activities	• Work with families to reduce the access of children to household cleaning products and medicines, by keeping them: – out of reach – in locked cupboards – in child-resistant packages – away from food and food containers • Work with families to increase supervision of children when near poisons • Encourage all families to remove and safely destroy all unneeded poisons and make sure poisons outside the house are locked away when not in use • Encourage families to clear places in and around the house where snakes, scorpions, and spiders can hide and breed • Educate families to wash work clothes that might be contaminated by poison, before letting them come into contact with other household contents or family members
Strategy 2	Increase the number of collaborative activities across the community designed to reduce risk factors for poison-related injuries and deaths
Activities	• Work with councils to: – create special poison-removal sites at dumps (rubbish tips) that are fenced away from public access – clear storage sheds in the village of poisons that could be found by people passing by – fence off or remove poisonous plants in the village streets – keep footpaths in the village well mown • Work with shop owners to store pesticides, detergents, and medications away from foods • Work with employers to: – make sure their workers wear protective clothing when spraying pesticides or insecticides in rural areas – make sure their workers follow the correct procedure when spraying insecticides and pesticides – make sure they do not release poisonous waste from their factories into the streets and rivers

<table>
<tr><td colspan="2" align="center">THE DINGLY POISONING PREVENTION ACTION PLAN</td></tr>
<tr><td>Our aim</td><td>To reduce hospitalizations and deaths from poisoning in Dingly by 10 per cent each year for the next five years</td></tr>
<tr><td>Strategy 3</td><td>Advocate to government and international aid groups to create and enforce poisoning prevention regulations</td></tr>
<tr><td>Activities</td><td>

• Create opportunities for the community to get involved in supporting legislative changes relating to:
  - the requirement for child-resistant closures on all poison, medication, and essential oil containers
  - accurate labelling of containers in which poisons and toxic substances are sold
  - readable descriptions and instructions on poison bottles (e.g. not written in small letters or another language)
  - workplace practices in relation to storage and use of poisonous substances

</td></tr>
</table>

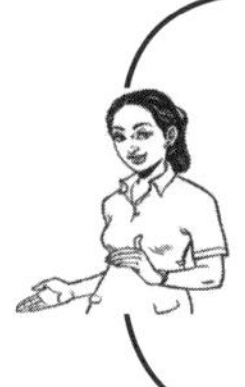

Help your group use the information they have gathered to identify what they must change to keep their community members safe. Use that discussion to develop a clear aim of the intervention. Work with your group to develop a poisoning prevention action plan for your community. Encourage your group to be clear about what risk factors they want to remove.

Putting the plan into practice

Dula's group started by showing the community it could manage the problem of poisoning. They focused on making changes that would become a part of everyday life.

Dula and the group visited the monthly meeting of the Women's Association of Dingly and discussed with them how to prevent poisoning at home. Members of the Women's Association came up with many helpful suggestions.

Dula and the group helped members of the Women's Association to organize a clean-up campaign in Dingly. They helped villagers to clean up around their houses and gardens, and advised on proper storage of harmful substances. They showed how to dispose of them safely once they were not needed.

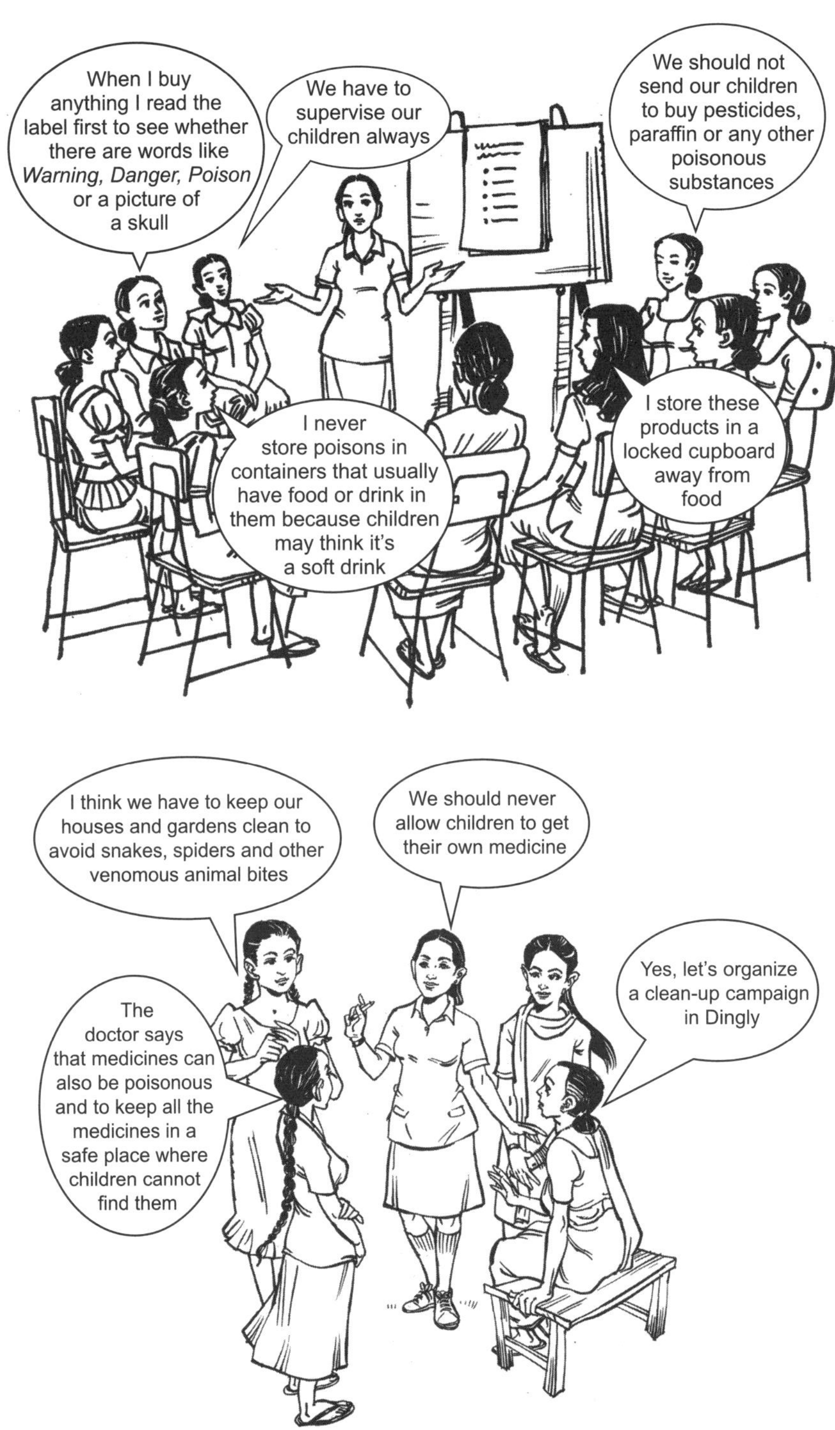

When I buy anything I read the label first to see whether there are words like *Warning, Danger, Poison* or a picture of a skull
We have to supervise our children always
We should not send our children to buy pesticides, paraffin or any other poisonous substances
I never store poisons in containers that usually have food or drink in them because children may think it's a soft drink
I store these products in a locked cupboard away from food
I think we have to keep our houses and gardens clean to avoid snakes, spiders and other venomous animal bites
We should never allow children to get their own medicine
The doctor says that medicines can also be poisonous and to keep all the medicines in a safe place where children cannot find them
Yes, let's organize a clean-up campaign in Dingly

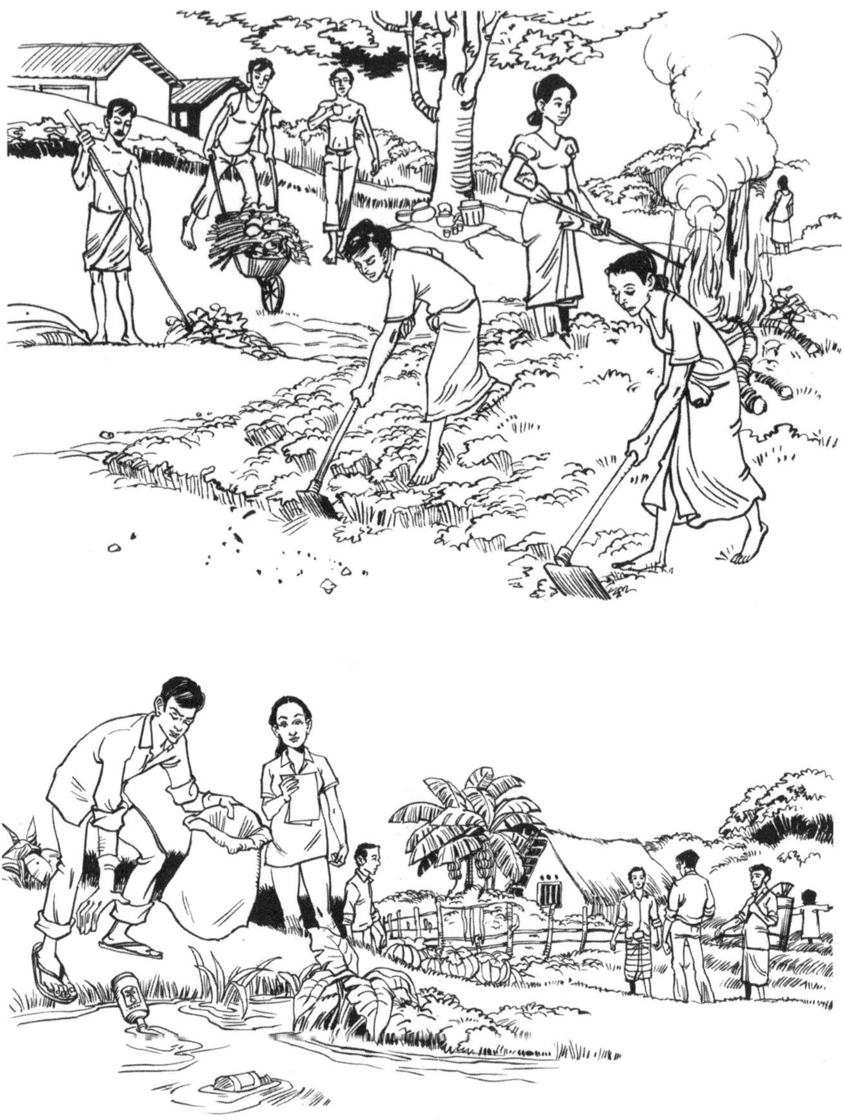

The Women's Association invited the villagers to a feast and a free movie at the community centre on the evening of the 'clean-up campaign' day. Dula borrowed a short video from the District Agricultural Department showing the correct ways of spraying pesticides, and the correct ways for safe storage, cleaning and discard of pesticide containers. Once most of the villagers and many farm owners were there, Dula started the movie.

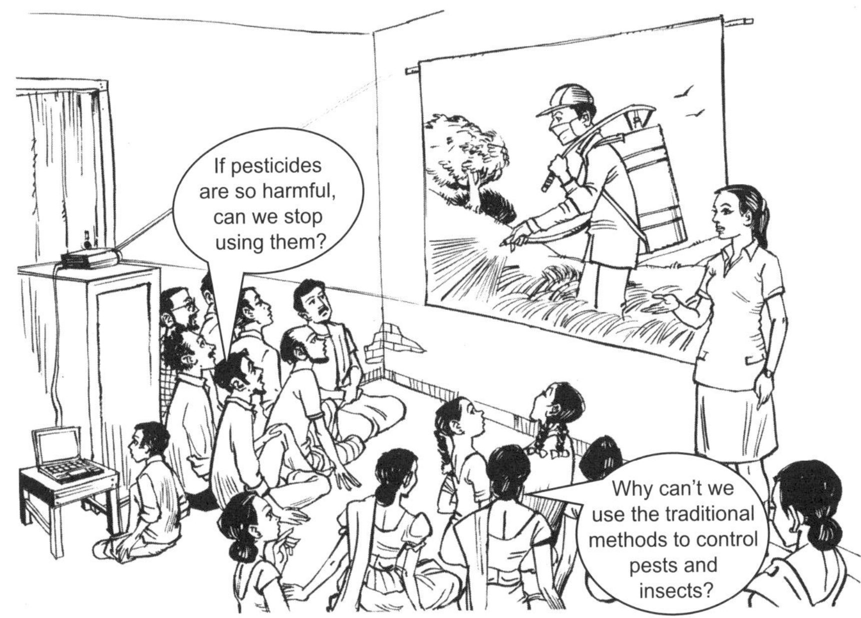

Dula had provided free pencils and paper to enable people to note down the following important messages about the use of pesticides:

- I have to wear protective clothing to cover my body completely.
- I should not spray on windy, rainy or cloudy days.
- It's better if I can spray in the early morning or late afternoon when it's not too hot.
- I should not touch my face, eyes and neck when spraying.
- While spraying, I should drink plenty of water after washing my hands.
- After spraying I must have a bath and wash my clothes before entering the house or touching my children.
- I have to wear gloves when washing my spray clothes and throw dirty water on *the field (never into any water body)*.
- I have to display the 'Do not enter' board in the field after spraying.
- I have to bury the empty pesticide container at least 50 metres away from any water source.
- I have to leave my crops for seven days before selling them or eating them.

Next steps

After watching the video on the clean-up campaign day, farmers had a lot of questions about pesticide poisoning.

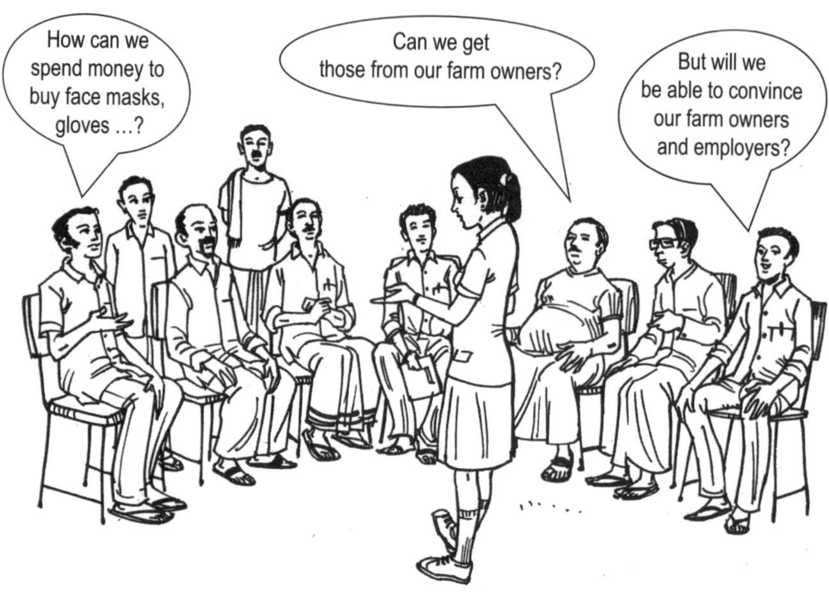

The Farmers' Alliance of Dingly asked farm owners to provide protective clothing and boots to all workers employed on their farms to prevent snake bites and poisoning through the skin or by inhaling poisonous vapours.

Dula and some members of the Employees' Trade Union of Dingly met with the employers to discuss steps they could take to prevent poisonings in their workplaces. They explained that healthy workers are good for business.

Some employers agreed to provide safety equipment and protective clothing to their workers when handling chemicals. They agreed to review the health and safety regulations and act as soon as possible to create a safe working environment for their workers. They asked Dula to conduct a workshop on poisoning for their workers. She invited a trainer from the health ministry to lead a practical training session demonstrating safety promotion and poisoning prevention activities in the workplace.

The group pressured shop owners in the village to store pesticides and other harmful substances away from food. They repeatedly wrote to the newspapers calling on the paper to print articles advising people across the community of the dangers of storing pesticides and other chemicals in the containers that can be opened easily by children.

As a result of their media campaign, one NGO gave out free containers with child-resistant closures to store these harmful household substances.

They started a 'wall magazine' at the community health centre. Dula encouraged people to post their drawings, poems, problems and suggestions about the poisoning problem and the solutions to the problem.

The working group wrote a letter to the government requesting a law to ban the chemicals that do not come in child-resistant containers. They further demanded that the instructions on how to use these chemicals be written on the containers in their own language. Most people in Dingly signed this letter before it was sent.

Dula and the group wrote a letter to the health minister requesting that the emergency care facilities in the Dingly Hospital be upgraded. They requested an increased annual supply of anti-venom and antidotes for the hospital.

The president of the Farmers' Alliance of Dingly wrote a letter to the pesticide manufacturers asking them to introduce child-resistant packaging to store pesticides. He frequently wrote to the local and national newspapers about the need for child-resistant packaging. Many people in Dingly decided not to buy detergents and other harmful substances that did not come in child-resistant packages.

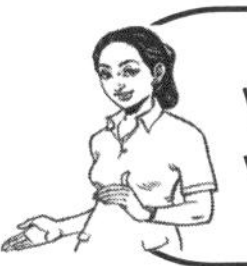

What can you learn from the way in which the poisoning prevention working group in Dingly put their action plan into practice?

As in most communities, women in Dingly are influential because they make decisions about their family's health, and they teach and care for the children. Initially, Dula reached out to the women in Dingly and convinced them of the need to address the problem of poisoning in Dingly. Then she educated the workers, who were mostly affected by this problem. They all planned and acted to change the community behaviour and modify their home and workplaces.

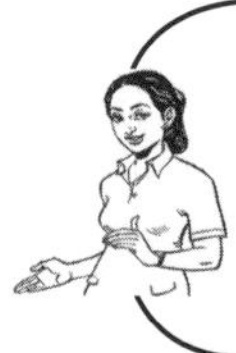

> What are the most influential groups in your community? Would they participate in changing the behaviour of your community to prevent death and injuries due to poisoning? What would be the barriers to approaching these groups? How could you overcome these barriers?

Progress monitoring

At the beginning of their implementation planning, Dula's group started to plan how they were going to know if all their hard work was making a difference.

The group knew that injury prevention programmes must be collaborative activities, with people from all over the community working alongside health promotion experts, scientists, and government members. The group felt that they needed to monitor what was done and the effects, and identify any other factors in the community that affected the way they were working.

They developed an intervention monitoring worksheet that they could complete to guide their planning.

The worksheet was four pages long. On the first page, they recorded information that would tell them whether the activities were implemented according to their plan. On the second page, they noted whether the desired changes in the community had been achieved. On the third page, they recorded information about whether the number and severity of injuries were decreasing. These questions were useful to monitor the effect of the strategies and to provide additional information that could be used to adapt the strategies as the needs of the community changed. On the fourth page, they collected data for the first six months and used the results to make adjustments to their implementation plan to improve its effectiveness. Dula's group repeated the evaluation at the end of the three years to measure the changes that had been achieved.

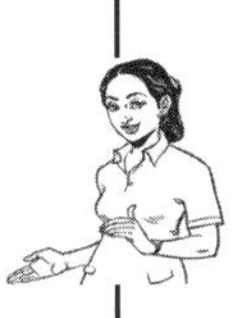

How will you monitor the interventions that you have implemented in your area? It is important to plan the monitoring process before you start your intervention. Talk through the various options with your group and decide how you plan to undertake the monitoring process.

In preparing the intervention monitoring process, ask your group to think about the following questions. What programmes will you undertake to prevent poisoning injury? What are the ways you will use to measure 'what is being done', 'what has changed', and 'changes in poisoning injuries that have resulted'? How are these changes being identified and recorded? Is there any information available from other sources that you could use in your evaluation?

Dula obtained the ethics approval and permission from relevant authorities before the group started collecting information from their community. Check with your local authority about what permissions you need.

MODULE 6
VIOLENCE

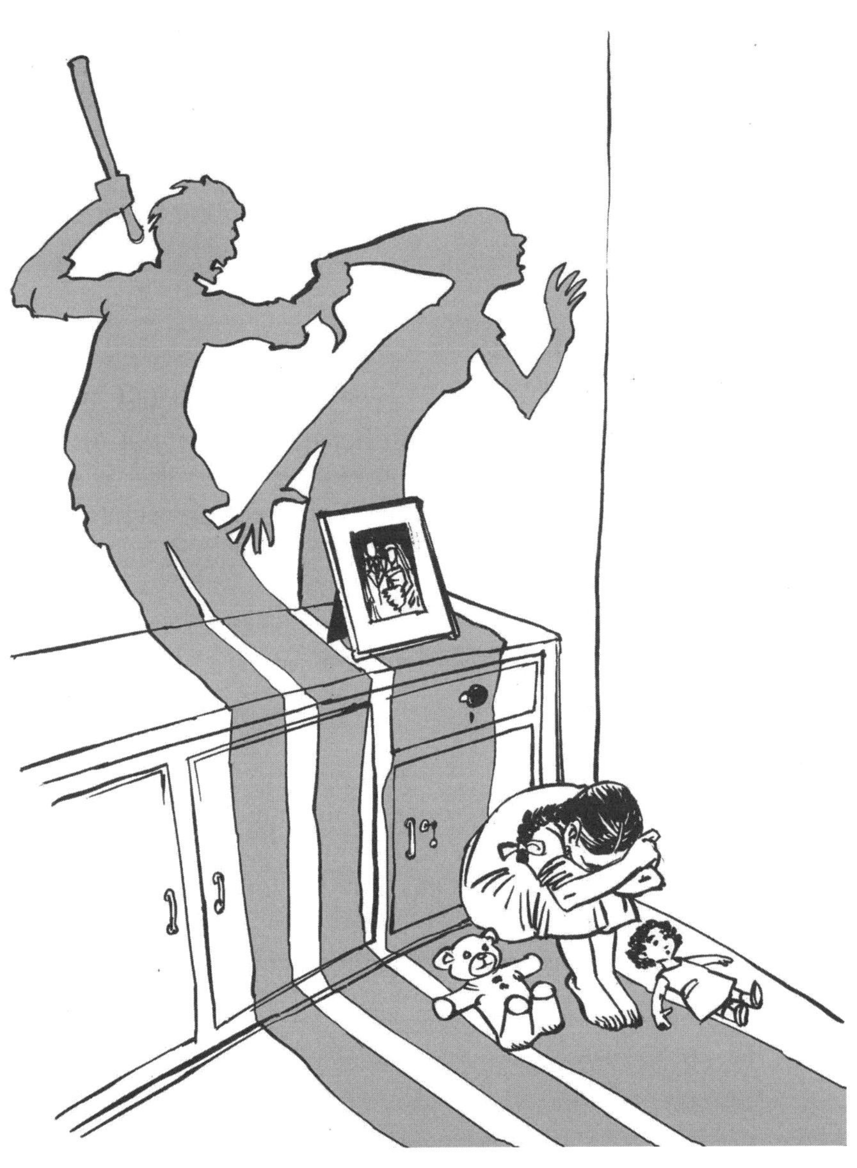

Violence-related injury is devastating. The causes of violence are complex but violence is preventable. Risk factors for violence include personal, neighbourhood and population-level factors. Underlying risk factors are particularly important in the causation of violence injury. This chapter provides a set of exercises to help you identify these factors. Once risk factors for violence injury have been identified, behavioural, environmental and regulatory changes can be made to address the factors and improve the safety of your community. The chapter looks at how violence prevention interventions can be developed and implemented, and explains how to develop an action plan for the reduction of violence in your community. You will also learn how to monitor the success of your plans.

Keywords: abuse, domestic violence, harm, intentional injury, stigma, violence prevention

Grasping the problem

Nadia was a 29-year-old mother of a preschool-aged child. She was found hanging from a bed sheet in her room when her drunken husband, Wazeer, came home late at night. Dula could remember her sorrowful face with a deep ragged scar running across her cheek. Wazeer had been beating her from the day after their marriage till her death.

Dula realized that violence was a major problem in Dingly but was not talked about because of embarrassment and fear. She was determined to put an end to it and raised the issue with the Injury Prevention Committee.

The committee decided to form a working group to find out more about the problem of violence-related injury in Dingly and to help the committee work towards making it totally unaccepted in Dingly. They invited representatives from the local council, religious leaders, police officers, health managers, the captain of the local cricket team, and the principal of the local school to be part of the working group.

http://dx.doi.org/10.3362/9781780448022.008

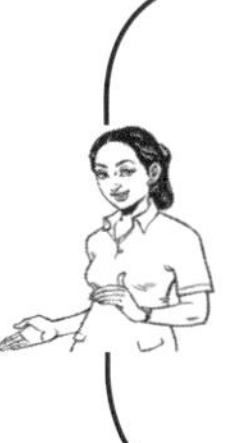

Do the members of your committee consider violence to be a problem in your community? Who are the people in your community who could help your committee develop and implement strategies to prevent it? Think widely and broadly about who could participate. Who will motivate the community to take action? Who will work to protect those who feel trapped in violent relationships? Invite these people to your next Injury Prevention Committee meeting to form a violence prevention working group.

What is violence?

Dula asked the group members to think for a few minutes about what they understood by the term 'violence'. She wrote their ideas on the board and used them to develop a definition of violence.

VIOLENCE

Violence is the purposeful use of physical force, power or words against oneself, another person, community or group. This can result in physical injury, psychological harm or death.

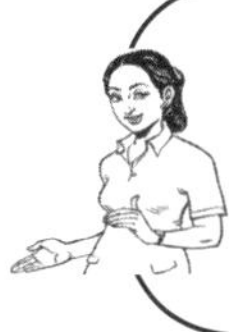

Tell a story like Nadia's to your group to set the scene for a discussion on violence. Remember not to use stories in which any individual or community could be known to the group. Then brainstorm with your group to find a definition of violence that is meaningful to the community your group is a part of.

Who can cause violence?

Dula's group felt the definition was accurate but did not give a true sense of all that happens when violence occurs. The complexity of meaning came out when the group explored the definition provided in more detail. To help support the group to express their feelings Dula wrote the beginning of a sentence on a flipchart and then each member of the group suggested a word to complete the sentence.

'Violence can be carried out by ...'

The whole group discussed their responses and put the people who they believed can commit violence into three broad groups.

Violence used by the individual (self-directed violence) against:

- themselves (self-harm, suicide);
- family members;
- children (child abuse);
- a spouse or partner;
- elderly parents or relatives (elder abuse).

Violence used by community members against:

- strangers;
- young people and children (bullying, slapping, punching, and threatening to use weapons);
- employees (employee abuse);
- prisoners.

Violence used by larger groups (collective violence):

- by states;
- by political groups;
- by terrorist groups.

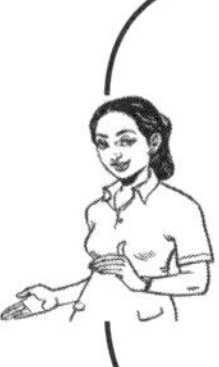

One of the ways you can help your group explore the meaning of violence is help them consider the range of people who are seen to be involved in violence, how the violence occurs, and who is harmed. This often helps people 'see' the range of situations where violence is used.

Ask your group to identify the people who can be involved in violence in your community.

How can they cause violence?

Dula and the group continued to explore the definition of violence at their next meeting. They focused this meeting on how people can cause violence.

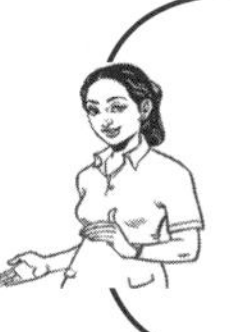

Talk with your group about different forms of violence. Ask your group to think about an example for each type of violence: physical violence, sexual violence, psychological violence, and neglect. Then make a list under each category of violence and discuss the examples your group put forward under each.

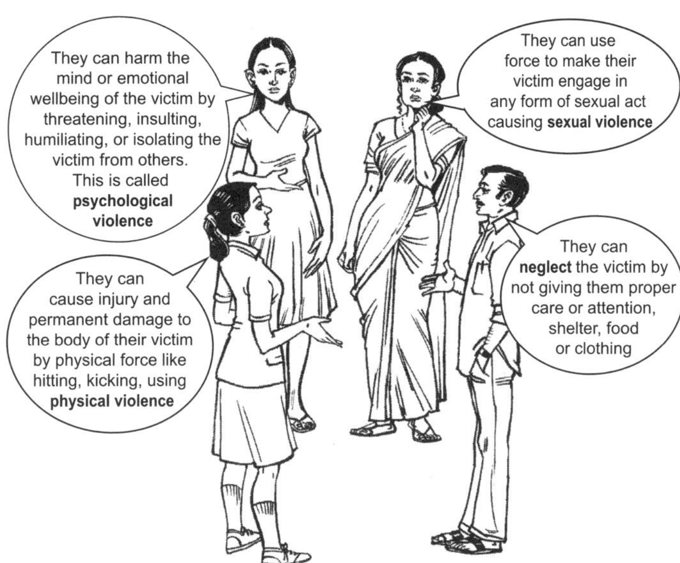

How can people be exposed to violence?

Violence is like a stone thrown into a pond. It strikes the water, but this immediate impact has a ripple effect that goes out to the far reaches of the pond. Violence in any part of a community can affect the whole community and future generations.

Dula's group discussed the level of exposure to violence.

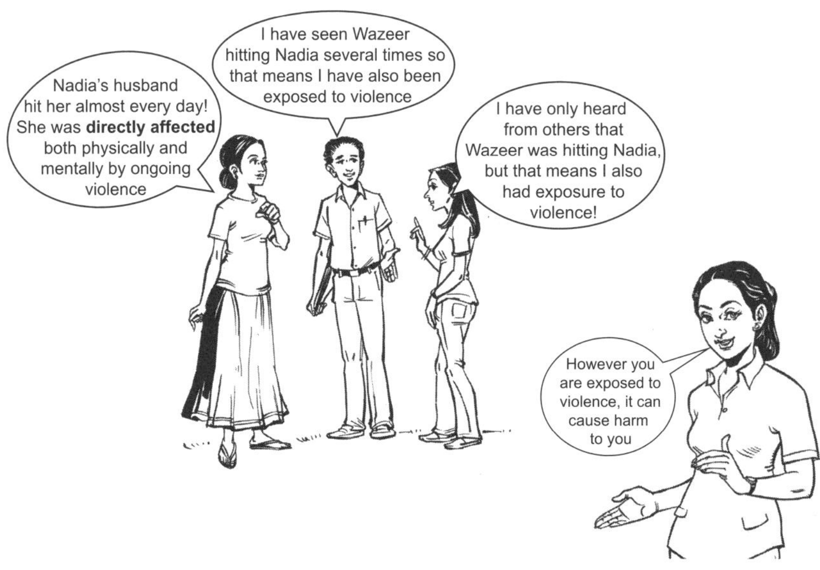

What are the outcomes of violence?

Violence can be devastating. It can be so bad that sometimes we try not to see what is happening because it distresses us too much. Dula's group was determined to take a frank and open look at the harm violence can cause so that they would be better equipped to deal with the problem in Dingly.

Dula divided her group into four smaller teams and nominated a narrator for each one. Then she gave one of the following stories to each team and asked them to discuss the outcomes they could see resulting from each story.

Story 1

Fifteen-year-old Lucy was an outstanding student in the class. Her class teacher had been sexually abusing and molesting her at the school for nearly six months. Her poor mother did not want to complain to the school administration fearing they would not believe Lucy. Now Lucy refuses to go to school and is having difficulty sleeping.

Story 2

A group of university students organized a meeting on the university campus to discuss the current political situation in the country. The police surrounded them and started shooting. Three students were shot dead and many others were injured.

Story 3

At the age of 17, Thashi watched as his father was killed right in front of him by a terrorist group. Since then he has wanted to get revenge. He joined a gang of young men involved in illegal activities so he could learn fighting skills.

Story 4

Thirty-two-year-old Fatima was dismissed from the garment factory after the birth of her first child. She had worked in this factory for the past 10 years.

When they had finished sharing ideas and experiences, the teams came back together and each narrator presented the summary of their group discussion to build a list of the possible outcomes from the violence described in each story. One group member summarized the main points on a flipchart.

Injured person

- pain;
- external injuries (cuts, lacerations, abrasions);
- broken bones;
- damage to nerves and brain;
- loss of appetite and poor nutritional status;
- developmental delay;
- poor performance at school or workplace;
- sexual dysfunction;
- sexually transmitted diseases;
- high-risk sexual behaviour;
- unwanted pregnancy;
- other reproductive health problems;
- mental health problems (depression, anxiety, self-harming, suicide);
- behavioural problems;
- poor interpersonal relationships;
- poor self-esteem;
- substance abuse (smoking, alcohol, drugs);
- loss of school or working days;
- unemployment;
- death.

Family members

- cost of treatment and rehabilitation;
- problems caring for the victim;
- loss of family income;
- not getting the care and support previously given by the victim;
- social stigma;
- victim may cause violence to others.

Community

- cost of treatment and rehabilitation of victims;
- property damage;
- fear and discrimination based on age or appearance;
- intolerance of different religions, cultures and customs;
- lack of opportunities provided for members of the community from different backgrounds to fully participate in community life.

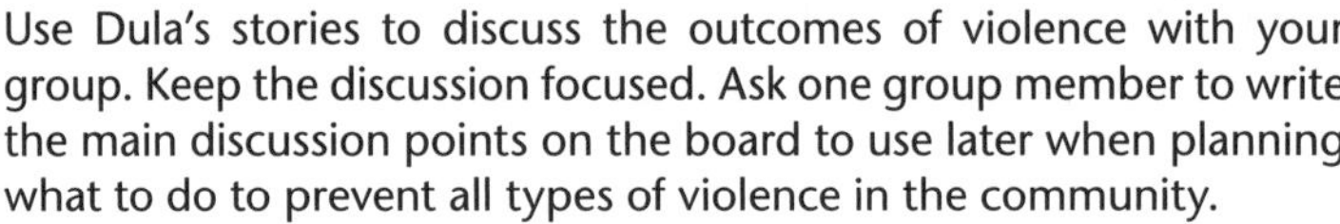

Use Dula's stories to discuss the outcomes of violence with your group. Keep the discussion focused. Ask one group member to write the main discussion points on the board to use later when planning what to do to prevent all types of violence in the community.

Some group members may be particularly sensitive to this discussion. Some may themselves have experienced violence. They may be acutely distressed by the discussion or may say things that make you realize they need help. Make sure you have a plan in place to refer these members of your group to the appropriate professional to provide the assistance they need.

Dula had a list of questions to help the group measure the nature and extent of the problem in Dingly: Who is being injured? Are the injuries to self or to others? Where are the injuries occurring? Are the injuries physical, emotional, or psychological? In what situations are these injuries occurring? How many people are often the victims of violence? How many people are often exposed to violence? Under what circumstances is violence happening? Are rates of violence changing over time?

The group quickly realized that this was going to be a much more difficult set of questions to answer than with other types of injuries. Information about violence is often hidden. People do not want to tell you. Nevertheless, the group developed a plan to get the answers they needed.

The main sources of information about how many, how often and how much damage was found at the clinics, health centres, hospital, and police station. However, the group was aware that police and hospital data does not give a true picture because victims often do not report violence or seek treatment for their injuries due to shame or fear of more violence.

To add to the bones of the information provided in the data, two female members of the group also conducted focus groups of women from the Women's Association of Dingly. Young male members went along to the schools, sports clubs and drinking places often visited by the men and boys of Dingly to gather information. Older members went to the village square and the Dingly Old People's Home to talk with the elderly people about their experiences of violence. Putting the available data and information gathered in the focus groups enabled the group to start building a picture of the size and nature of the problem in Dingly.

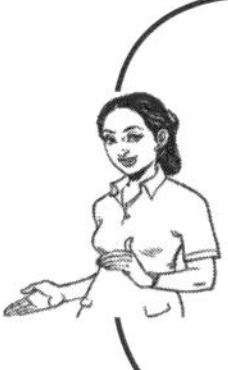

Go through the same process with your group to work out the size and nature of the problem in your community. Which groups of people are more at risk of violence by others? Which groups are using violence against others? Which groups are at risk of self-harming? When and where is violence happening? What injuries are occurring?

Risk factor identification

Dula divided the group into four small teams and asked each team to identify individual-, family-, neighbourhood-, and population-level risk factors for violence. Once they had talked about what they already knew, she asked them to write down questions they did not have answers to. She told the group that she would try to find out the answers to their questions.

Before the next meeting, Dula did a lot of work searching for the answers. She spoke to the violence prevention NGOs and to the government ministries responsible for child welfare, and human services. She went to the findings that had been written down in library books and on the internet.

At the next meeting of the working group Dula reported back, and the group continued to discuss the issues. At the end of this session, Dula summarized their discussion in a list.

Individual- and family-level risk factors for violence

- exposure to violence;
- substance abuse (alcohol and other drugs);

- unequal distribution of power and responsibilities between family members;
- exposure to high levels of family stress;
- poor social interactions within the family/community;
- lack of individual and family communication and problem-solving skills;
- availability of weapons.

Neighbourhood-level risk factors for violence

- social inequality;
- unemployment;
- lack of social support for families;
- power structure within the village;
- community beliefs;
- lack of reporting of acts of violence;
- lack of education;
- lack of opportunities for different groups to participate equally in community events;
- stigma associated with being a victim of violence;
- lack of community interactions.

Population-level (structural) risk factors for violence

- differences in the valuing of community members according to gender, social, ethnic, racial, religious, or economic status;
- lack of the rule of law;
- poor enforcement of public violence laws;
- disruption of modern social structures and community functioning caused by historical social/cultural/political/economic injustices.

At the end of this meeting, Dula realized the group was having trouble properly understanding how the risk factors were related to people being intentionally harmed. So she arranged for a series of presentations to the working group by experts from the social welfare groups to explain common risk factors for each type of violence in more detail.

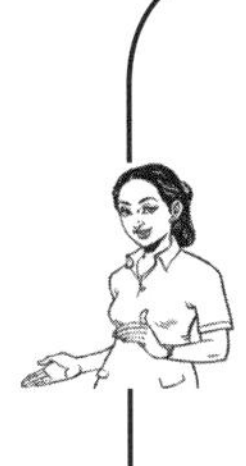

Conduct a group discussion to identify risk factors for violence in your area. Pay particular attention to the underlying causes of violence at each level: individual, neighbourhood, population. You may need to get help from experts to come up with the full range of answers needed by your group to empower them to find solutions. Visits by experts will help people understand better how the risk factors for violence contribute to harm in your community. Spend time with your group explaining each of the issues involved. The solutions will be stronger and longer lasting, and will protect more people if you take the time now to look at the issues from all viewpoints.

Intervention development and implementation

Setting aims for interventions

The working group for violence prevention in Dingly was formed and realized quickly that they had a difficult job. However, the group strongly believed that it was important to reduce the problem of violence in Dingly. In fact, it was essential if Dingly was to grow and prosper as a place where people could live full and productive lives.

So they could focus their efforts, the group agreed on a clear aim for their violence reduction activities. They decided they wanted *'to reduce hospitalizations and deaths from violence in Dingly by 10 per cent each year for the next three years'*.

Dula's group drafted an action plan for discussion with the whole village (see next page).

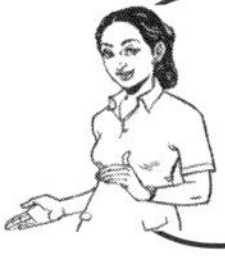

Work with your group to set aims for the interventions you plan to implement to reduce the injuries and deaths caused by violence in your area.

THE DINGLY VIOLENCE PREVENTION ACTION PLAN	
Our aim	To reduce hospitalizations and deaths from violence in Dingly by 10 per cent each year for the next three years
Strategy 1 *Activities*	Build understanding across the community about the causes of violence-related injuries and deaths in Dingly • Work with community groups in encouraging families to reduce unequal distribution of power and responsibilities between family members • Support families to build their understanding of the importance of good social interactions within the family • Support girls to go to school for as long as possible • Encourage aid organizations to provide low-interest loans to women to enable them to build their self-esteem through starting their own small business • Conduct workshops at the schools and at the Baby Health Clinic to help women and girls understand what help is available if they are victims of violence • Conduct workshops in schools, workplaces, factories, and farms to teach men and young boys that violence in any form is unacceptable and will not be tolerated • Support people to report acts of violence
Strategy 2 *Activities*	Increase the number of collaborative projects across the community designed to bring people of all cultures and backgrounds together • Work with governments, councils, employers, and community services to build tolerance and standards of acceptable behaviour by creating opportunities for all members of the community to live, work and play together • Encourage people from all social and cultural backgrounds to participate in the power structure within the village • Provide a safe place for victims of violence and resources to meet their immediate daily needs

Strategy 3
 	
Activities
	Advocate to government and international aid groups to create and enforce violence prevention laws across the community
	
	• Create opportunities for the community to get involved in creating social change to ensure:
	  – equality in the way people of different gender, social, ethnic, racial, or economic status are valued
	  – respect for the rule of law
	  – repair of the damage done to social structures and functions caused by past injustice
	  – reduced availability of weapons

Putting the plan into practice

Dula's group talked about how they would put their violence prevention action plan in place. After a lot of discussion and sharing of ideas, the group agreed that they would begin by using a street drama festival to raise awareness of the problem.

Dula prepared some storylines and asked the group members to make up short plays about acts of violence. Some of the storylines they acted out are listed below.

- An elderly mother has to do all the housework of her son's family.
- A 12-year-old girl has to care for her young siblings after the death of her mother. Her father is not sending her to school.
- A woman raped by a stranger is now pregnant and her husband has chased her from their home.
- An employer in the village is exploiting his workers by making them work long hours for very poor pay.

The group members developed the scripts and played different roles. Most of the people in Dingly came to the drama festival and watched the plays with knowing eyes and much nodding of the head. Dula group members were sitting in the audience to encourage everyone to talk about the difficulties that each character in the stories faced. In this way, the wall of silence around violence in the community began to break down.

Next steps

Dula and the group started to talk about violence with all parts of the community. They visited the school, the hospital, the church, the temple, the mosque, and other religious places to talk about violence. At all times they made sure they were aware of and sensitive to the culture of the group they were meeting with. They were careful not to cause further intolerance or division within the community.

The Women's Association, the youth club and the factory workers' trade union invited them to their regular meetings. Dula went on the local radio station to talk about the problem of violence in Dingly and steps that every person living in Dingly could take to help reduce the risk of violence to them and to others.

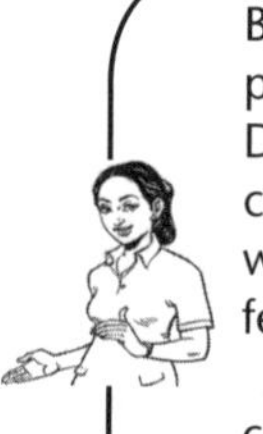

By inviting representatives from the local council, religious leaders, police officers, health managers, and other resource groups in Dingly, Dula had built relationships with the people who had the capacity to address the problem of violence. The fact that violence was being talked about openly helped reduce the fear and shame felt by many victims of violence.

What activities can you carry out to raise awareness in your community that all forms of violence cannot be tolerated? How will raising this awareness help you implement your violence prevention activities?

Next, the group decided to work to improve interactions between people in the community. They organized a New Year festival in the village in collaboration with the youth club. Local council members, traders' associations, NGOs, and charity groups sponsored this event. Families in Dingly came with their children and enjoyed a variety of activities. The organizing committee hoped the festival would become an annual event to nurture community tolerance and strengthen feelings of belonging to the one community among the people who lived in Dingly.

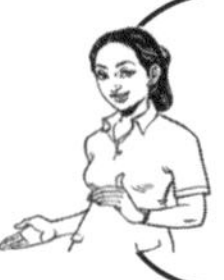

Are there other activities that you can think of to improve interactions within your community? How could you organize them? What are the resources you can use? What will be the barriers to organizing these activities? How are you going to overcome these barriers?

Dula and her group organized workshops on parenting and life skills to be held regularly in the village community centre. She arranged for professionally trained facilitators to attend the meetings to talk about how acceptance of violence starts in the family. The topics included positive parenting, importance of early childhood care, developing coping skills, and stress management. Professional staff from the child health and community centre discussed ways to support victims of violence. Parents were encouraged to discuss with other group members the difficulties they faced with caring for their children, and facilitators were able to suggest solutions for their problems.

Dula's group also identified other opportunities to address the problem. They worked with clinics to improve child services and care for pregnant mothers, and established parent support groups in the community. They promoted activities at schools outside normal school hours, and vocational training programmes for school leavers.

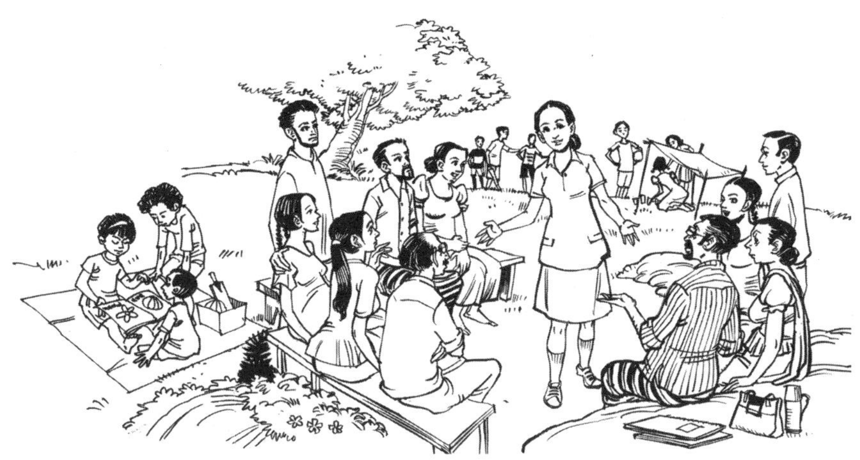

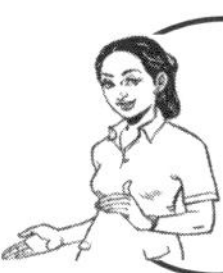

Encourage your group to think of activities to prevent violence towards children and young people in your area.

Dula encouraged the youth club of Dingly to launch a 'stay safe with alcohol' campaign. They displayed posters in the village marketplace about the advantages of not misusing alcohol and other addictive substances. The group developed interventions to discourage alcohol advertising and the illegal production of alcohol in the village. They developed a range of options about how alcohol in the community could be regulated in a way that decreased alcohol abuse and alcohol-related violence. They developed support groups for people who were dependent on alcohol and drugs, and worked with welfare and clinical treatment agencies to improve funding for appropriate management.

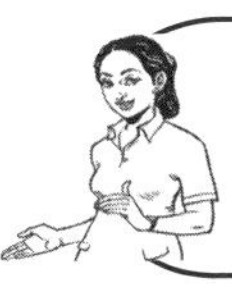

What activities could you carry out to establish an alcohol-free environment in your area?

The group realized that they could help address the causes of violence in their community by increasing people's access to resources. When the village women were employed, they not only earned money and thus had more independence, but they also had a greater confidence and self-esteem. The meaningful employment of women and young girls helped to distribute power and responsibility equally between men and women in the family and the community.

The group arranged a series of workshops on self-employment. Speakers from several government departments were invited to conduct training sessions. The group encouraged people in Dingly to make use of their skills such as sewing and knitting to earn an income. They worked with the local bank to establish a small loan system with easy payment schedules to help the members of the community to buy basic equipment needed for their projects.

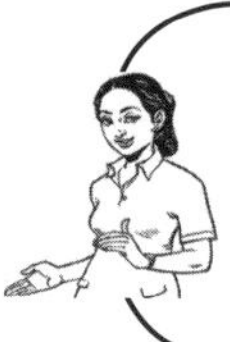

As community workers, we can educate and guide our community on the available resources such as banking facilities, self-employment opportunities, small-scale industry, and apprenticeship programmes. Are there other activities that could improve employment of women and young girls in your area?

Dula and her group organized a health camp for elderly people in the village. Doctors were invited to screen the elderly for diseases such as diabetes, high blood pressure, and heart disease. Care givers were encouraged to come to the camp with their elderly family members. The religious leader of the village visited the camp and gave a talk on the value of caring for the elderly. They established senior citizens' associations to build opportunities for social interactions and to promote active participation in community events and decision-making.

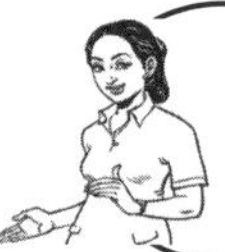

How could your group start to address the problem of violence toward older people in your community?

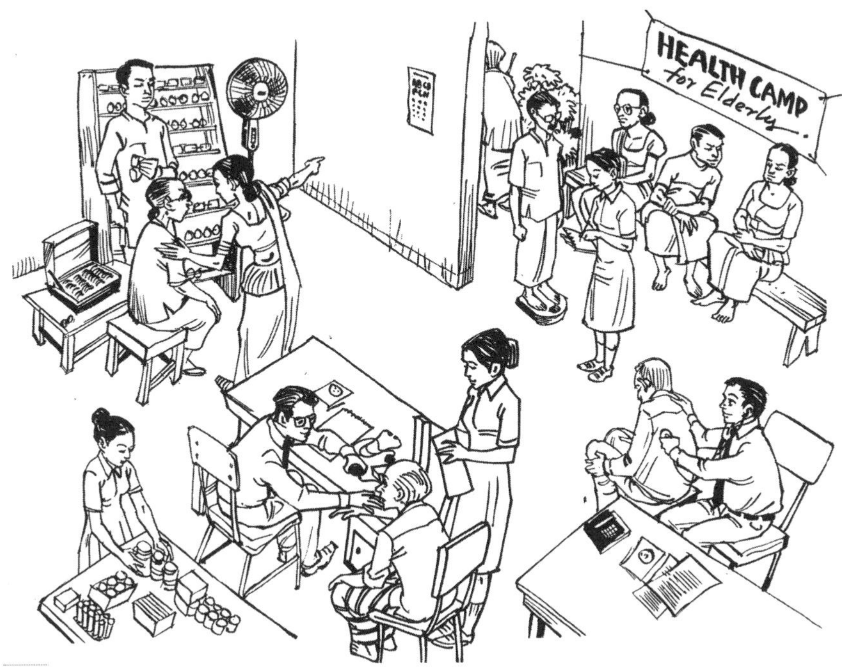

Representatives from the group arranged to meet with the state minister. Before the meeting, Dula prepared a brief letter in which she described the problem of violence in Dingly, and outlined some of the possible solutions identified by looking at the information gathered by the group. During the meeting, the group members asked for the minister's support to help the community begin to address the community acceptance that promoted violence in Dingly.

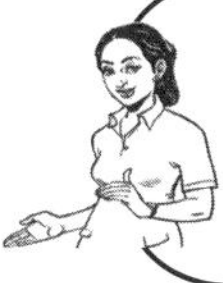

Could your group convince the politicians of your community to take action to prevent violence-related injuries and deaths? What will be the barriers for communicating with the politicians? How can you overcome them?

Progress monitoring

Dula and the group planned to evaluate the intervention programmes to make sure they were working as well as they had planned. They wanted to find out three main things: Were the activities being implemented as they had intended? Were the desired changes in the community being achieved? Did these changes result in fewer violence-related hospitalizations and deaths?

They had developed an evaluation plan at the same time as they had developed their intervention plan. Progress against the goals was recorded on an intervention monitoring worksheet for each of their interventions over the past twelve months.

The worksheet was four pages long. On the first page, they recorded information that would tell them whether the activities were implemented according to their plan. On the second page, they noted whether the desired changes in the community had been achieved. On the third page, they recorded information about whether the number and severity of injuries were decreasing. These questions were useful to monitor the effect of the strategies and to provide additional information that could be used to adapt the strategies as the needs of the community changed. On the fourth page, they collected data for the first six months and used the results to make adjustments to their implementation plan to improve its effectiveness. Dula's group repeated the evaluation at the end of the three years to measure the changes that had been achieved.

Using these worksheets, Dula's group was able to report on the success of their violence prevention plan. They also had good information to help improve their strategies of into the future.

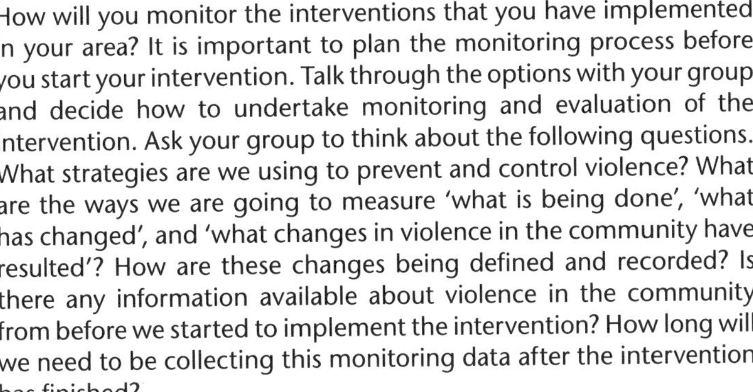

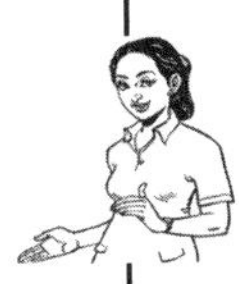

How will you monitor the interventions that you have implemented in your area? It is important to plan the monitoring process before you start your intervention. Talk through the options with your group and decide how to undertake monitoring and evaluation of the intervention. Ask your group to think about the following questions. What strategies are we using to prevent and control violence? What are the ways we are going to measure 'what is being done', 'what has changed', and 'what changes in violence in the community have resulted'? How are these changes being defined and recorded? Is there any information available about violence in the community from before we started to implement the intervention? How long will we need to be collecting this monitoring data after the intervention has finished?

Dula obtained the ethics approval and permission from relevant authorities before the group started collecting information from their community. Check with your local authority about what permissions you need.

MODULE 7
OTHER INJURIES

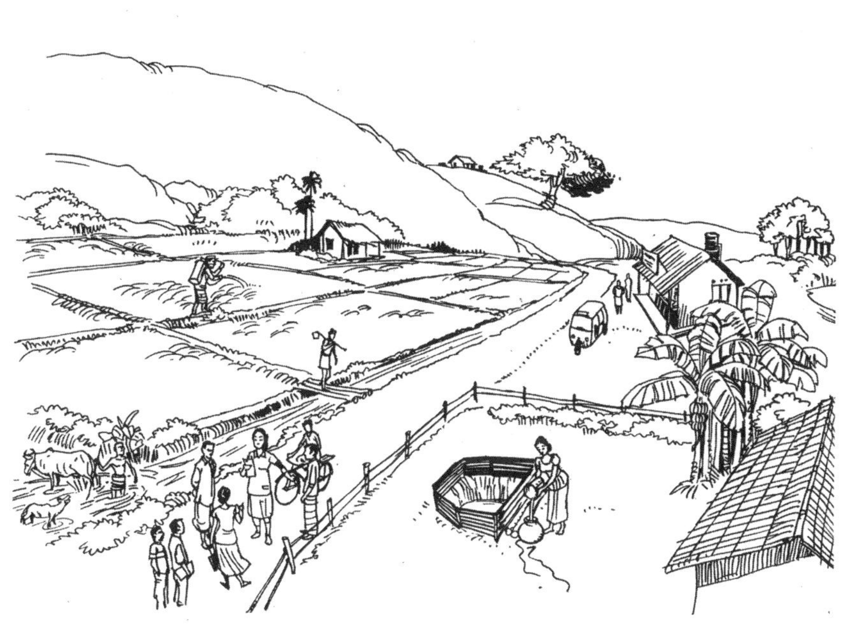

This module presents a generic approach you can use in your community to prevent injury from any cause. The easy way to remember this approach is to think of the word GRIP. G stands for Grasping the problem, R stands for Risk factor identification, I stands for Intervention development and implementation, and P stands for Progress monitoring. For any type of injury you want to address, all you need to do is follow the guidelines for these four steps, and you will be able to help reduce the problem in your community.

Keywords: action plans, injury prevention, interventions, progress monitoring, risk factors, surveillance

One day Dula and members of the Injury Prevention Committee walked around the village to look at how well their injury prevention activities were working. Most people in Dingly were using safe oil lamps and safe stoves. They had fixed guards over the windows and fences around the wells. They were using child-resistant containers to store harmful substances.

But they met a farmer attacked by a bull. He had several injuries to his back and legs. A three-year-old girl had crushed her fingers in a door when her brother closed it. A 16-year-old boy had twisted his ankle when playing football.

They realized that there are lots of different ways to be injured that still needed to be addressed.

At the next Injury Prevention Committee meeting, Dula asked everyone to name all the injuries that they could think of that were not burns, falls, drowning, transport, poisonings or violence-related injuries. One committee member wrote their responses on the flipchart. They grouped them into categories to create this list:

- bites, scratches, attacks by animals;
- being crushed by falling objects ;
- fingers, hands or arms being cut or crushed in machines;
- explosive blast injuries;
- sports injuries.

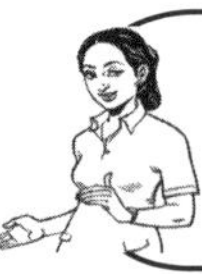

Talk with your Injury Prevention Committee about other injury types they have experienced and that could be addressed.

http://dx.doi.org/10.3362/9781780448022.009

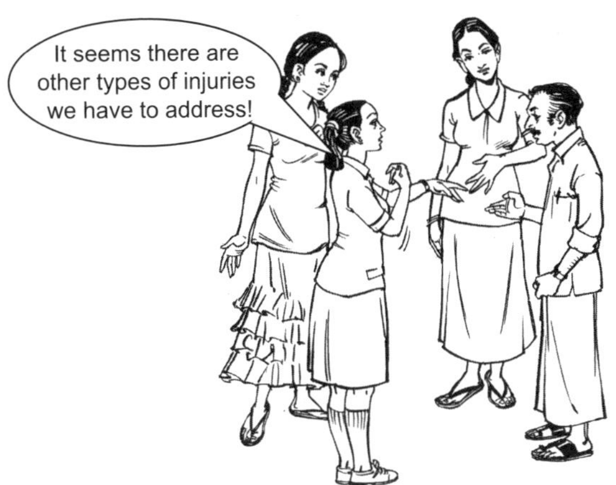

It seems there are other types of injuries we have to address!

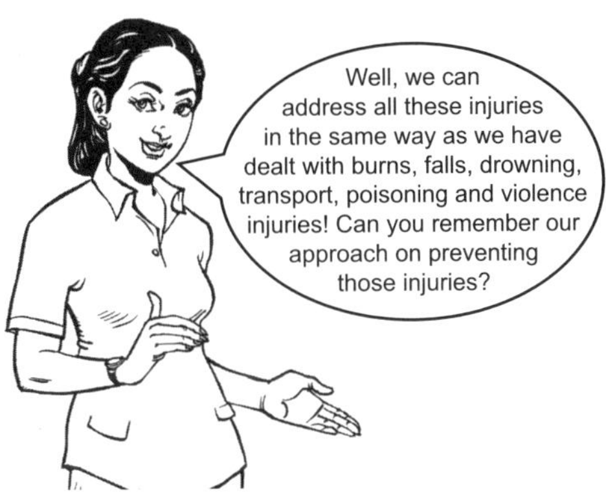

Well, we can address all these injuries in the same way as we have dealt with burns, falls, drowning, transport, poisoning and violence injuries! Can you remember our approach on preventing those injuries?

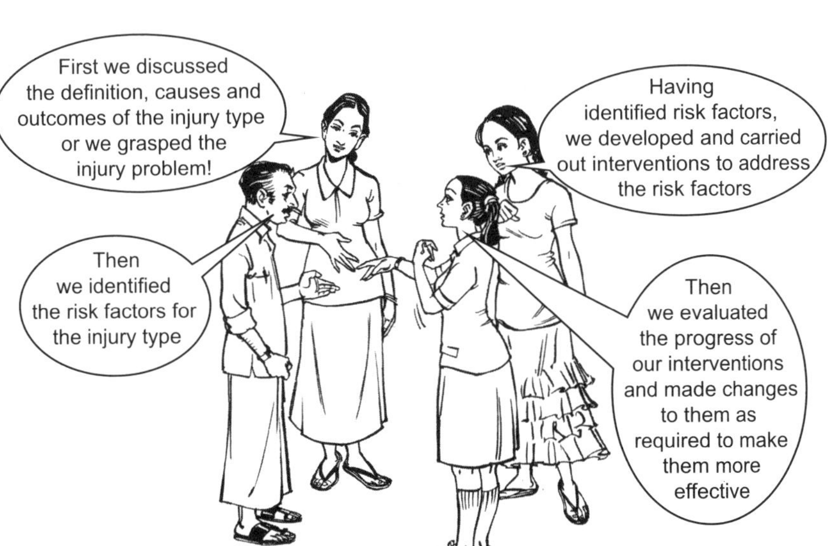

First we discussed the definition, causes and outcomes of the injury type or we grasped the injury problem!
Having identified risk factors, we developed and carried out interventions to address the risk factors
Then we identified the risk factors for the injury type
Then we evaluated the progress of our interventions and made changes to them as required to make them more effective

Dula's committee recognized the four-step approach to addressing any injury type they could come across in Dingly.

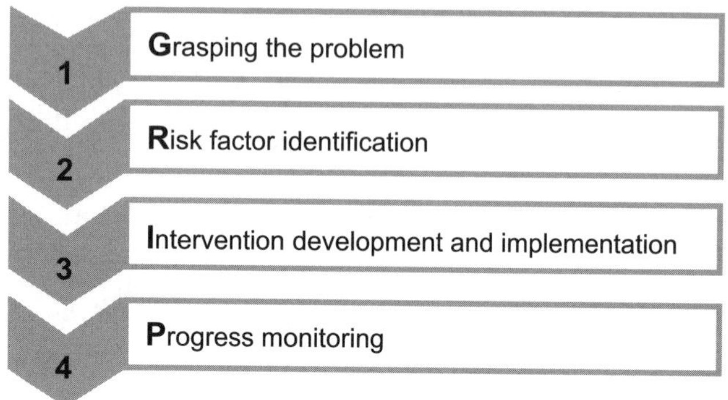

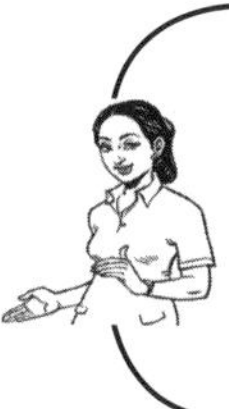

Talk with your committee about using the pattern they have been following for their response to each of the injury problems in *The GRIP Guide*. Work with them to understand how this four-step approach can be used as a guide for addressing any other injury type they may come across. Use the following sections of this module to illustrate how useful the four-step approach can be.

Grasping the problem

After all the work the Injury Prevention Committee had done, they had become experienced injury prevention practitioners. They found it easy to identify the questions they needed to ask in order to understand a 'new' injury, whatever it might be. After a brief discussion, the committee wrote up these questions on a board:

- What energy is involved?
- How does the energy transfer take place?
- Which body part is damaged?
- What is the damage?
- Where does the injury occur?
- What activity are the injured people doing when the injuries occur?
- What are the consequences of the injury for the individual, the family, and the community?

These questions provide information that can be used to plan injury prevention activities in your community.

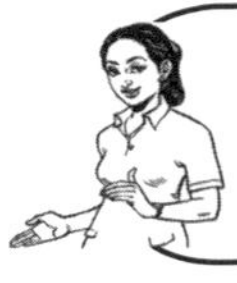

Ask your committee members to describe the types of injury they have identified in their community.

Dula explained that the process of 'grasping the problem' is the same as 'identifying the nature and extent of the problem' or 'describing the epidemiology of the problem'. Injury surveillance, like other forms of health surveillance, can provide an ongoing source of information for injury prevention. She asked her committee to list the possible sources of such information.

The committee remembered some of the places they had gone to find information for their interventions to prevent burns, falls, transport injuries, drowning, poisoning, and violence. These sources could be used to obtain information about any sort of injury. They collected their ideas and summarized them on the blackboard:

- police records;
- hospital or emergency department records;
- school records;
- workplace accident records;
- community surveys;
- mass media;
- publications;
- focus group discussions with community members.

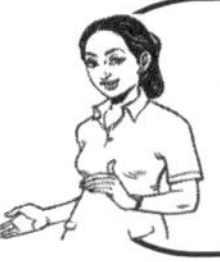

Talk with your group about how they could set up an ongoing routine injury surveillance system using existing data sources.

Risk factor identification

Individual, family, neighbourhood and population level

Dula asked her committee members to think about the methods they had used to identify risk factors for burns, falls, drowning, transport injuries, poisoning, and violence. After some discussion the committee summarized these on a flipchart.

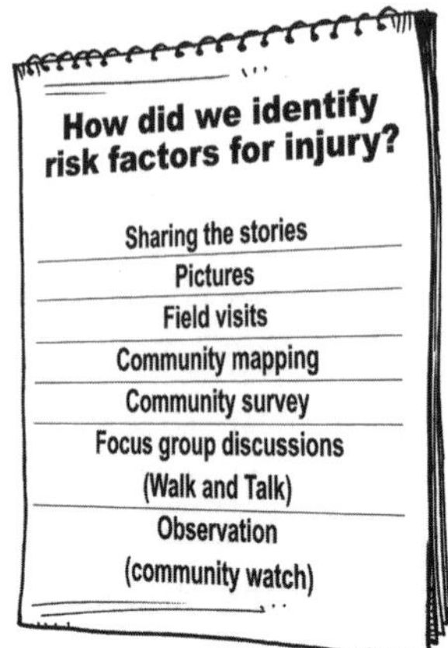

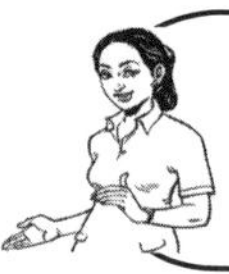
Can your group think of other methods to identify the risk factors for injuries?

Dula's committee also constructed a risk factor table as shown in Table 7.1 that they could use for any type of injury they chose. Whenever they approached a new injury problem all they needed to do was list the risk factors they identified against the points in the section the risk factors related to.

Table 7.1 Risk factors at different levels

Level of operation of risk factor	Risk factors
Individual/family level	•
Neighbourhood level	•
Population level	•

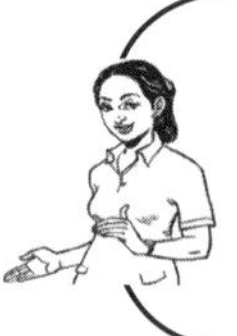
By analysing the causes of injury in your community according to a risk factor table, you can plan injury prevention activities more effectively. To help your committee understand how to use this table, ask them to think of some of the risk factors for the new injury types they identified earlier and summarize them in the table.

Intervention development and implementation

Setting aims for interventions

Once an injury problem and its risk factors have been described, the next thing to do is to set aims for interventions. The way to start is to describe what you want to be different after the intervention.

The aim should be sustainable, measurable, achievable, realistic, and time-specified (SMART). Then go on to develop an action plan. An action plan lists activities that need to be completed for the aim to be effective.

Dula divided the committee into five small teams and asked each to set aims for interventions to prevent one of the injury types identified earlier in this module:

- bites, scratches, attacks by animals;
- being crushed by falling objects;
- fingers, hands, or arms being cut or crushed in machines;
- explosive blast injuries;
- sports injuries.

One member of each team presented the summary of their team's discussion to the whole committee. The committee then developed a general approach to setting aims for interventions that they could apply to any injury, regardless of the type of injury it was.

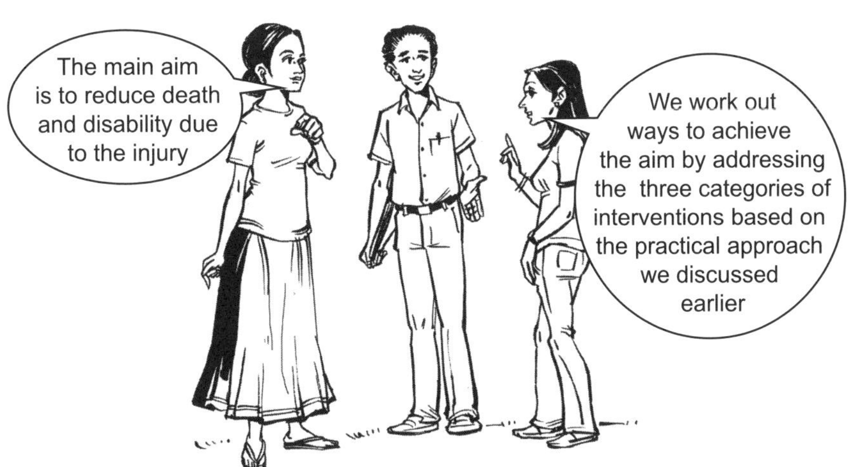

Dula's group came up with a guide to help them prepare interventions to prevent the injury type they identified as a priority.

Our main aim

- To reduce injuries and deaths due to ______________ injury by ______________ per cent per year in Dingly

How can we achieve this aim?

- Change the behaviour of people in Dingly to prevent ______________ related deaths and injuries

- Modify the environment in homes and the community to reduce ______________ related deaths and injuries

- Encourage political leaders to set up rules and guidelines to prevent deaths and injuries due to ______________

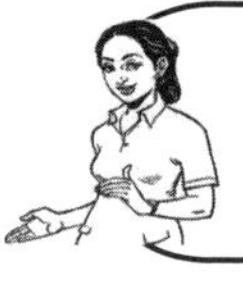

Repeat Dula's exercise with your committee.

Prioritizing

Dula's Injury Prevention Committee was now able to understand the problem of injury as a health condition that had many component parts but which all followed the same principles of causation and prevention and management.

It was clear to the committee that there was much that could be done to address the problem of injury in Dingly. The question they had was: where do you start?

The committee followed the approach they had learnt and practised. They divided into teams and listed the criteria they considered when deciding which injuries in Dingly needed to be addressed first. One member summarized the thoughts of the whole committee on a flipchart.

What factors to consider when prioritizing the other injury types that need to be addressed?

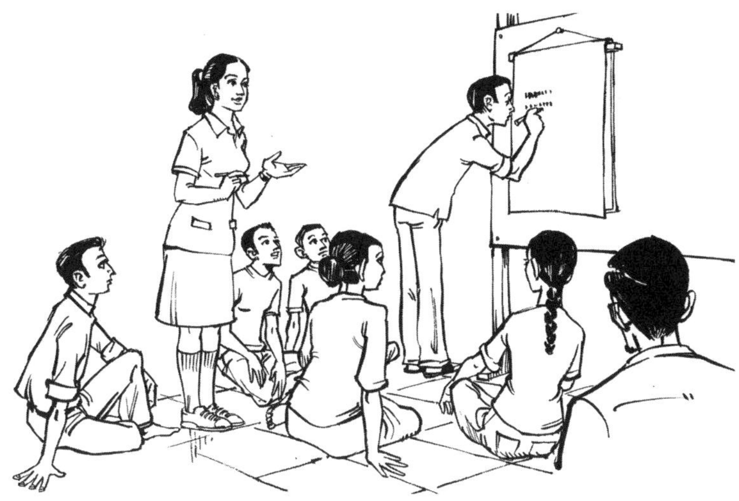

- How frequent is the injury? Example: injuries due to dog bites occur more frequently than injuries following earthquakes in Dingly.
- How severe is the injury? Example: injuries following contact with an operating machine are more severe than a cut injury with a cooking knife.
- What is the risk group involved? Example: injuries to children may need more attention.
- Are there any successful, low-cost interventions in other communities? Example: there may be ways to fence and cover wells that have been used in other communities.
- Can our community afford the interventions? Example: fencing off a water channel may be possible even if installing pipes is too expensive.
- Are the interventions culturally acceptable? Example: the type of clothing that needs to be worn to be safe can be adapted to suit what is acceptable for the community.
- Are the interventions in line with government policies and the legal system? Example: ways to encourage workplaces to introduce safety measures can be adapted to fit within legal requirements.

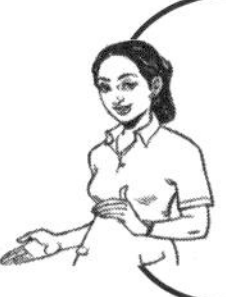

Work with your committee to develop criteria to be considered when prioritizing injuries that need to be addressed in your community? Ask your committee to prioritize what they should do next to address the problem of injury in your community.

Putting the plan into practice

Now that Dula's committee had developed a general approach that would work for whichever injury type they chose to address, they now needed a general way of thinking about how they could put their interventions into practice.

Dula asked her committee members to form small teams to discuss this next challenge, then report back to the group and compare their ideas. One member of the committee summarized the final discussion on the board.

What are the issues we have to think when putting injury prevention interventions into practice?

- What is the target group the intervention is aimed at? Examples: school children, old people, young people.
- Where are we going to carry out the intervention? Examples: schools, homes, workplaces.
- What have others done to address the same injury? Examples: success stories from other communities.
- Are the interventions suitable to our community? Examples: culture, beliefs, community structure, facilities available, level of education.
- How are we going to modify the interventions to suit our community? Examples: local expertise, locally available less-expensive materials, local regulations and processes for supporting safe behaviour.
- Are there several interventions to address one injury type at the same time? Examples: educate the people, make changes in the environment, enforce laws, and make policy changes.
- Do we have the resources to carry out the interventions? Examples: people, funding.

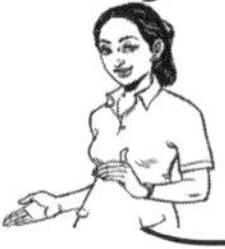

Talk with your committee about the issues you will need to think about when developing injury prevention interventions in your community.

Progress monitoring

The final part of the GRIP process is performance monitoring. Dula asked her committee members to talk with a person sitting near them about what this means. She asked each pair to complete the following sentence on a piece of paper: 'We monitor the progress of injury prevention programmes because we want to ...'

Here are some of their answers:

- determine whether the activities are carried out according to the plan;
- determine whether the community is accepting the interventions;
- determine whether the programme is achieving the aims of the interventions;
- determine ways to improve the interventions;
- make the community more confident that the interventions are of benefit.

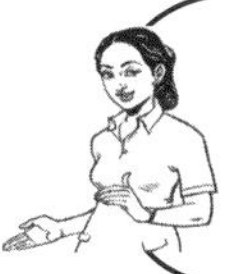

Start the discussion on monitoring injury prevention programmes with your committee using the techniques Dula used. Ask your committee members to think of more reasons to monitor injury prevention programmes implemented in your community.

When and how to monitor progress?

Dula and the committee talked about the importance of developing a project evaluation plan at the beginning of the project. For any new injury problem, they could think through the issues of progress monitoring at the same time as they were developing a project implementation plan.

They also talked about the importance of data collection sheets that could be used to collect information to monitor progress. These progress monitoring information sheets could be completed at the beginning of the project, then regularly (for example, six-monthly) over the period of the programme implementation. They developed a template that described the general approach they could follow to create a project evaluation plan for any future injury programme.

Project evaluation plan

1. What is the intervention?

2. What is the objective?
    –   Who will be changed?
    –   What do we need to change?
    –   Where do we expect to change?
    –   How would we measure the change?
    –   How many will change?
    –   When do we expect this change to occur?

3. When to monitor?
    –   before the intervention;
    –   mid-way;
    –   after the intervention.

4. How to monitor?
    –   questionnaire, survey, checklist;
    –   interviews;
    –   observation;
    –   focus groups.

5. What kind of information do we need?
    –   Can people afford the intervention?
    –   Can people access the intervention?
    –   Can people maintain the intervention?
    –   Are there any problems with the intervention?
    –   Other useful information?

6. Who will collect information?

7. How will we collect information?

8. How will we analyse the information?

9. Who to report the results to?

10. What is the next step?

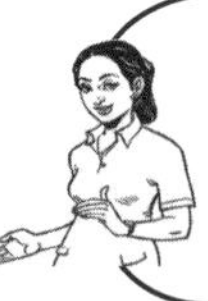

Talk with your committee about the methods they might use for monitoring the injury prevention interventions. See if they can create some templates they could adapt for use to monitor the success of injury prevention projects they introduce.

CHAPTER 3

Putting it all together

The prevention of injuries involves working with the community to:

- count the number of injuries;
- identify the causes of the injuries;
- work out the best ways to correct the causes;
- make sure that as many of these causes as possible are corrected.

When developing solutions, it is important to be aware of how the intervention is likely to be used, who by, and in what environments. Interventions need to be appropriate to the values and practices of the target population and be acceptable.

The aim of any intervention should be sustainable, measurable, achievable, realistic, and time-specified (SMART).

Ultimately, the usefulness of the methods we implement to correct the causes of injury is determined by how they are used in the community. The effectiveness of the implementation requires the community to work together at the grass roots level, with commitment from the social and political structures and institutions that support the community growth.

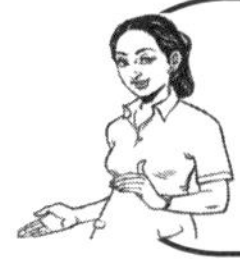

Check with your local authority about ethics approval and permission from relevant authorities before the group starts collecting information from their community.

Dula's working group is only just starting on their journey of solving the problem of injury in Dingly. What they have done is not the only way of doing things; you may see ways of doing it better for your community. What they have done well is to demonstrate a process you can use to help you develop your own solutions.

The GRIP Guide helps you 'learn by doing', not 'do by copying'. Now is your chance to continue to help your community solve the problem of injury where you live.

http://dx.doi.org/10.3362/9781780448022.010

Bibliography

Arshi, S., Sadeghi-Bazargani, H., Mohammadi, R., Ekman, R., Hudson, D., and Djafarzadeh, H. (2006) 'Prevention oriented epidemiologic study of accidental burns in rural areas of Ardabil, Iran', *Burns* 32: 366–71.

Celis, A. (1997) 'Home drowning among preschool age Mexican children', *Injury Prevention* 3: 252–6.

Conant, J. and Fadem, P. (2008) *A Community Guide to Environmental Health*, Berkeley, USA: Hesperian Foundation.

David, F. and Duncan, P.H. (1996) 'Growing up under the gun: children and adolescents coping with violent neighborhoods', *Journal of Primary Prevention,* 16 (4): 343–56.

Dharmaratne, S.D. and Ameratunga, S.N. (2005) 'Road traffic injuries in Sri Lanka: a call to action', *Journal of the College of Physicians and Surgeons Pakistan* 14 (12): 729–30.

Dharmaratne, S.D. and Stevenson, M. (2007) 'Public road transportation in a low income country', *Journal of the International Society for Child and Adolescent Injury Prevention* 12 (6): 417–20.

Doan, S. (2008) 'Health-seeker level workshop report, Binghampton', Memphis, TN: Memphis Religious Health Assets. <http://mrhap.fatcow.com/binghampton_seeker.pdf> [accessed June 2013].

Forjuoh, S. (2003) 'Traffic-related injury prevention interventions for low income countries', *Injury Control and Safety Promotion* 10: 109–18.

Forjuoh, S.N. (2006) 'Burns in low- and middle-income countries: a review of available literature on descriptive epidemiology, risk factors, treatment, and prevention', *Burns* 32: 529–37.

Haddon, W. (1970) 'On the escape of tigers: an ecologic note', *American Journal of Public Health and the Nation's Health* 60 (12): 2229–34.

Haddon, W. (1980) 'Advances in the epidemiology of injuries as a basis for public policy', *Public Health Reports* 95 (5): 411–21.

Hahm, H. and Guterman, N. (2001) 'The emerging problem of physical child abuse in South Korea', *Child Maltreatment* 6: 169–79.

Holder, Y., Peden, M., Krug, E., Lund, J., Gururaj, G., and Kobusingye, O. (eds) (2001) *Injury Surveillance Guidelines*. Geneva: World Health Organization (WHO).

Hope, A. and Timmel, S. (1995) *Training for Transformation: A Handbook for Community Workers,* Books 1–3, Rugby, UK: Practical Action Publishing.

Hope, A. and Timmel, S. (1999) *Training for Transformation: A Handbook for Community Workers,* Book 4, Rugby, UK: Practical Action Publishing.

Hyder, A.A., Borse, N.N., Blum, L., Khan, R., El Arifeen, S. and Baqui, A.H. (2008) 'Childhood drowning in low- and middle-income countries: urgent need for intervention trials', *Journal of Paediatrics and Child Health* 44: 221–7.

Krug, A., Ellis, J., Hay, I., Mokgabudi, N., and Robertson, J. (1994) 'The impact of child resistant containers on the incidence of paraffin (kerosene) ingestion in children', *South African Medical Journal* 84 (11): 730–4.

Krug, E.G., Dahlberg, L.L., Mercy, J.A., Zwi, A.B., and Lozano, R. (eds) (2002) *World Report on Violence and Health*, Geneva: WHO.

Marsh, D., Sheikh, A., Khalil, A., Kamil, S., Jaffer-uz-Zaman, Qureshi, I., Siraj, Y., Luby, S., and Effendi, S. (1996) 'Epidemiology of adults hospitalized with burns in Karachi, Pakistan', *Burns* 22: 225–9.

Mathie, A. and Cunningham, G. (2003) 'From clients to citizens: asset-based community development as a strategy for community-driven development', *Development in Practice* 13 (5): 474–86.

Matteucci, M.J., Hannum, J.E., Riffenburgh, R.H., and Clark, R.F. (2007) 'Pediatric sex group differences in location of snakebite injuries requiring anti venom therapy', *Journal of Medical Toxicology* 3: 103–6.

Matzopoulos, R. and Carolissen, G. (2006) 'Estimating the incidence of paraffin ingestion', *African Safety Promotion: A Journal of Injury and Violence Prevention* 3: 4–14.

McClure, R. (2010) 'Injury risk and prevention in context', *Injury Prevention* 16 (6): 361–2.

McClure, R.J., Hughes, K., Ren, C., McKenzie, K., Dietrich, U., Vardon, P., Davis, E., and Newman, B. (2010) 'The population approach to fall injury prevention in older people: findings of a two community trial', *BMC Public Health* 10: 79 <http://dx.doi.org/10.1186/1471-2458-10-79>.

McClure, R., Stevenson, M. and McEvoy, S. (eds) (2004) *The Scientific Basis of Injury Prevention and Control*, Melbourne, Australia: IP Communications.

National Crime Prevention Centre (2000) *A Manual for Community-Based Crime Prevention: Making South Africa Safe*, Pretoria: CSIR.

Nordberg, E. (2000) 'Injuries as a public health problem in sub-Saharan Africa: epidemiology and prospects for control', *East African Medical Journal* 77 (12 Suppl): S1–43.

Ozanne-Smith, J., Day, L., and Parsons, B. (2001) 'Childhood poisoning: access and prevention', *Journal of Paediatrics and Child Health* 37: 262–5.

Parry, C.D.H. and Dewing, S. (2006) 'A public health approach to addressing alcohol related crime in South Africa', *African Journal of Drug & Alcohol Studies*, 5 (1): 41–56.

Peden, M., McGee, K., and Krug, E. (eds) (2002) *Injury: A Leading Cause of the Global Burden of Disease*, Geneva: WHO.

Peden, M., Oyegbite, K., Ozanne-Smith, J., Hyder, A.A., Branche, C., Fazlur Rahman, A.K.M., Rivara, F. and Bartolomeos, K. (2008) *World Report on Child Injury Prevention*, Geneva: WHO.

Pinkett, R. (2000) 'Bridging the digital divide: sociocultural constructionism and an asset-based approach to community technology and community building', paper presented at the 81st Annual Meeting of the American Educational Research Association (AERA), New Orleans, LA, April 24–28. <http://alumni.media.mit.edu/~rpinkett/papers/aera2000.pdf> [accessed June 2013].

Rahman, A., Giashuddin, S.M., Svanström, L., and Rahman, F. (2006) 'Drowning – a major but neglected child health problem in rural Bangladesh: implications for low income countries', *International Journal of Injury Control and Safety Promotion* 13: 101–5.

Reza, A., Krug, E.G., and Mercy, J.A. (2001) 'Epidemiology of violent deaths in the world', *Injury Prevention* 7: 104–11.

Rotary International (n.d.) *Community Assessment Tools. A Companion Piece to Communities in Action: A Guide to Effective Service Projects*, Evanston, IL: Rotary.

Samarakkody, D., Gunathunga, W., and McClure, R. (2009) 'Influence of child care pattern and behaviour on unintentional injuries among preschool children', *Proceedings of the 9th National Conference on Injury Prevention and Safety Promotion*, p. 51, Melbourne, Australia: Monash University Accident Research Centre.

Samuel, N., Forjuoh, S.N., and Gyebi-Ofosu, E. (1993) 'Injury surveillance: should it be a concern to developing countries?' *Journal of Public Health Policy* 14 (3): 355–9.

Seedat, M. (1999) 'The construction of violence in South African newspapers: implications for prevention', *Peace and Conflict: Journal of Peace Psychology* 5 (2): 117–35 <http://dx.doi.org/10.1207/s15327949pac0502_2>.

Seedat, M., Van Niekerk, A., Jewkes, R., Suffla, S., and Ratele, K. (2009) 'Violence and injuries in South Africa: prioritizing an agenda for prevention', *Lancet* 374: 1011–22.

Sethi, D., Habibula, S., McGee, K., Peden, M., Bennett, S., Hyder, A.A., Klevens, J., Odero, W. and Suriyawongpasisal, P. (eds) (2004) *Guidelines for Conducting Community Surveys on Injury and Violence,* Geneva: WHO.

Sharma, P.N., Bang, R.L., Al-Fadhli, A.N., Sharma, P., Bang, S., and Ghoneim, I.E. (2006) 'Paediatric burns in Kuwait: incidence, causes and mortality', *Burns* 32: 104–11.

Sherker, S., Short, A., and Ozanne Smith, J. (2005) 'The in situ performance of playground surfacing, implications for maintenance and injury prevention', *International Journal of Injury Control and Safety Promotion* 12 (1): 63–6.

Spiegel, C.N. and Lindaman, F.C. (1995) 'Children can't fly: a programme to prevent childhood mortality from window falls', *Injury Prevention* 1 (3): 194–8.

Spinks, A., Turner, C., McClure, R., Acton, C., and Nixon, J. (2005) 'Community based programmes to promote use of bicycle helmets in children aged 0-14 years: a systematic review', *International Journal of Injury Control and Safety Promotion* 12 (3): 131–42.

Spinks, A., Turner, C., Nixon, J., and McClure, R.J. (2009) 'The "WHO Safe Communities" model for the prevention of injury in whole populations (Review)', *The Cochrane Library* 2009 (3) <www.thecochranelibrary.com/ userfiles/ccoch/file/Safety_on_the_road/CD004445.pdf> [accessed May 2013].

Storoschuk, S. (2001) *Injury Prevention Program Evaluation Manual*, Vancouver, BC: British Columbia Injury Research and Prevention Unit.

Svanstrom, L. (2012) 'It all started in Falköping, Sweden: Safe Communities – global thinking and local action for safety', *International Journal of Injury Control and Safety Promotion* 19 (3): 202–8.

Svanstrom, L. and Haglund, B.J.A. (2000) *Evidence-based Safety Promotion and Injury Prevention: An Introduction,* Sundbyberg, Sweden: Karolinska Institute.

Turner, C., McClure, R., Nixon, J., and Spinks, A. (2004) 'Community based programmes to prevent pedestrian injuries in children 0–14 years: a systematic review', *International Journal of Injury Control and Safety Promotion* 11 (4): 231–7.

Turner, C., McClure, R., Nixon, J. and Spinks, A. (2005) 'Community based programs to promote car seat restraints in children 0–16 years: a systematic review', *Accident Analysis and Prevention* 37: 77–83.

United States Department of Health and Human Services (2001) *Youth Violence: A Report of the Surgeon General,* Washington, DC: Office of the Surgeon General.

Wallace, L.J.D. (2002) *Evidence-Based Effective Strategies for Preventing Injuries: Child Restraints, Seat Belts, Reducing Alcohol-Impaired Driving, Teen Drivers, Child Abuse Prevention, Bike Helmets, Residential Fire, and Drowning,* National Center for Injury Prevention and Control, Atlanta, GA: Centers for Disease Control and Prevention.

Werner, D., with Thuman, C. and Maxwell, J. (2011) *Where There Is No Doctor: A Village Health Care Handbook,* Berkeley, CA: Hesperian Health Guides.

World Health Organization (WHO) (1996) 'Violence: a public health priority', WHO Global Consultation on Violence and Health, Geneva: WHO.

WHO (1999) *WHO Multi-country Study on Women's Health and Domestic Violence,* Geneva: WHO.

WHO (2002) *Injury Prevention and Control in the South-East Asia Region,* Report of an Intercountry Consultation, Bangkok, Thailand, 23–26 January 2002, VIP, New Delhi: WHO <http://whqlibdoc.who.int/searo/2002/SEA_Accidents_7.pdf> [accessed June 2013].

WHO (2004) 'How can injuries in children and older people be prevented?', Denmark: WHO Regional Office for Europe Health Evidence Network <www.euro.who.int/__data/assets/pdf_file/0004/74686/E84938.pdf> [accessed June 2013].

WHO (2007) *International Statistical Classification of Diseases and Related Health Problems, 10th Revision,* Geneva: WHO.

WHO (2008) *Falls,* Violence and Injury Prevention and Disability project, Geneva: WHO.

WHO (2012) 'Training, educating and advancing collaboration in health on violence and injury prevention (TEACH-VIP 2): users' manual', Geneva: WHO <http://whqlibdoc.who.int/publications/2012/9789241503464_eng.pdf> [accessed June 2013].

WHO and International Society for Burn Injuries (2006) *Facts about Injuries: Burns,* Geneva: WHO.